Osseointegrated Dental Technology
Graham E. White

Osseointegrated Dental Technology

Graham E. White, M Med Sci., PhD., CGIA.

Dental Instructor, University of Sheffield
School of Clinical Dentistry, Sheffield England

Director, University of Sheffield
Dental Advice Research and Technology Service

Former Chief Examiner in Dental Technology,
City and Guilds of London Institute

Quintessence Publishing Co Ltd.
London, Berlin, Chicago, and Tokyo

First published 1993 by
Quintessence Publishing Company Ltd
London, UK

British Library Cataloguing—in Publication—Data

White, Graham
Osseointegrated Dental Technology
I.Title
617.6

ISBN 1-85097-031-9

Lithographed, printed and bound in Jurong
(Singapore) by Toppan Printing Co. (S) Pte. Ltd.
from typesetting by av-Satz, Berlin (Germany)

Contents

Preface   11
Foreword   12
Acknowledgements   13
Dedication   14
Glossary of Special Terms Used   15

Chapter One
Introduction   19
The Brånemark dental implant   20
The use of implants   20
Sheffield dental technology and research   24
Osseointegrated implants   24
Osseo-disintegration   24
Team-work   25
Training   25
Persistent Precision Provides Predictable Prognosis   26

Chapter Two
Laboratory Equipment   27
Magnification   28

Chapter Three
The Installation of Implants   31
Pre-surgical treatment planning   31
Drilling stents   32
Fixture installation   36
Temporary prostheses   38
Abutment connection   39
Implant positions   43
Failure of fixtures to osseointegrate   44
The technical significance of fixture loss replacement   44

Chapter Four
Provisional Prostheses   47
Temporary prostheses   47
Intermediate prostheses   48
Novice prostheses   48

The construction of temporary and intermediate prostheses   48
   The single tooth
   Sheffield clips
Temporary components   51
   Temporary cylinders
The construction of a bridge for the EsthetiCone abutment   53
   Temporary tubes
Construction of a cemented temporary bridge   56
   Installation
Construction of screw retained prostheses with cast frameworks   57
Construction of a single tooth using the temporary cap   58

Chapter Five
The Design of Frameworks for Complete Prostheses   61
The Sheffield fitting test   61
Framework design   61
Safe bearing   62
Framework materials   62
Principals of framework design   62
   Fixture length and bone quality
   Masticatory loads
Analysis of masticatory loads   63
   Skalak/McGuire theorem
   Finite element analysis
   Castigliano's theorem
   Conclusions
Gold screw pre-load   66
Casting alloys and investments   67
   Control of alloy temperature
   Melting type 4 gold alloys
   Results
      Experienced technicians
      Inexperienced technicians
   Metal-ceramic alloys
   Results
   Conclusions
   The choice of alloy for frameworks
Casting investments   71
Strengthening heat treatment   72
The fatigue resistance and strength of Sheffield frameworks   72
   Fatigue resistance
   Strength
Framework fitting accuracy   75
Misfitting frameworks   76

Passively fiting one—piece frameworks
Aspects of osseo-disintegration   78
   Horizontal framework misfitting
   The effect of horizontal framework misfitting
The connection accuracy of gold screws and gold cylinders   82
   Results
The significance of replica errors   85
The fracture and loosening of gold screws   86
An improved abutment replica for the Brånemark implant   90
Abutment replicas from independent manufacturers   90
Conclusions   90
Factors which may affect the long—term survival of osseointegrated
dental implants   92

Chapter Six
Angulated Abutments   **95**
The function and use of angulated abutments   97

Chapter Seven
The Construction of a Mandibular Fixed Complete Framework   **103**
Primary impressions — study casts   104
Special tray construction   104
Impression materials   104
Placement of abutment replicas   104
The re-use of components   108
Framework construction   108
Pattern making   108
   Resin sub-frame
   Addition of wax
Pattern strain relief   115
Spruing the pattern   115
Ring lining   117
Mould orientation marker for centrifugal casting   117
Pattern preparation   117
Investments   118
Investing and mould heating   118
Amount of casting metal required   120
Pre-casting mould cooling   121
Strengthening heat treatment   121
The fit of frameworks   123
Framework finishing   124
Recording framework dimensions   126
Final fitting inspection   127
Framework try-in and jaw registration   129

Chapter Eight
Setting-up and Finishing Fixed Complete Prostheses   **133**
Trial dentures   *134*
Method 1   *134*
  Advantages of method 1
  Disadvantages
  Setting-up the teeth
Method 2   *138*
  Advantages of method 2
  Disadvantages
  Setting—up the teeth
Screw access holes   *140*
Try-in of dentures and finishing   *142*
Processing   *145*
  Grinding-in the occlusion
  Polishing
Fitting the prosthesis   *149*
Archiving completed work items   *151*

Chapter Nine
Overdentures   **153**
Denture instability   *153*
Designing overdentures for functional stability   *153*
Tooth positioning for functional stability   *154*
  Analysis of denture bearing foundations
The construction of implant supported lower and conventional complete
upper prostheses   *154*
Tooth materials   *156*
Setting-up the teeth   *156*
Overdenture retention systems   *157*
Type 1 retainers   *159*
  Articulated retention grip bars
    Dolder bars
  Dolder bar joint
  Overdenture kit with gold bar
    Cast bar
    Wrought bar
Type 2 retainers   *166*
  Ball attachment
Incorporating retention systems in dentures   *166*
Processing and finishing   *166*
  Grinding-in the occlusion

Chapter Ten
The Construction of Maxillary Fixed Complete Prostheses   169
Prostheses with resin teeth   169
Metal-ceramic prostheses   171
Selection of metal-ceramic materials   172
   Gold cylinders
   Casting alloy and porcelain
The construction of compound metal-ceramic prostheses   172
   Pattern making
   Investing, casting and finishing
   Fitting the prosthesis
Prostheses with anterior cantilevers   179

Chapter Eleven
The Partially Dentate Mouth   185
Treatment planning   186
The CeraOne abutment and crown   186
   The construction of ceramic CeraOne crowns
   Metal-ceramic CeraOne crowns
   The fit of metal-ceramic CeraOne crowns
Partial prostheses   193
Prostheses with resin teeth   195
The EsthetiCone abutment   195
   Fixture position
The construction of metal-ceramic prostheses using EsthetiCone abutments   197
The fitting of prostheses   199

Chapter Twelve
Maintenance and Repairs   203
The replacement of worn acrylic teeth and denture base   205
Fracture of denture base resin   205
Fractured overdenture clips   205
   Fractured clips and curved bars
   Nobelpharma Overdenture Kit type DCA 110
   Nobelpharma Overdenture Kit type DCA 130
      Clip problem 1
      Clip problem 2
      Clip replacement
Fractured overdenture bars   209
Distorted and fractured frameworks   209
   Distorted frameworks
   Fractured frameworks
Broken gold screws   215

The repair of prostheses containing obsolete parts   *216*
   Conical gold screws and matching cylinders
   Single tooth abutment

Chapter Thirteen
Treatment Consequences   221

Chapter Fourteen
Technical Data   225

Index   231

Preface

Professor Per-Ingvar Brånemark has provided dentistry with a very special gift indeed. That by using his methods many patients who previously had the most intractable prosthetic problems now have the prospect of long–term treatment success is astounding. Reliable procedures are now available which offer a treatment option for virtually every extent and pattern of tooth loss.

Dental technology plays a crucial part in this achievement. Although conventional technology and clinical dentistry can be adapted to implant work, much of this will be inappropriate for implant supported prostheses.

A different approach is needed for many aspects of implant dentistry.

This book is written for those dentists and dental technicians whose interests centre on providing prostheses which are specifically designed to be supported by implants. The main methods and materials described are those determined by dental technology research followed by extensive clinical use.

Words do not exist to express the distressful shortcomings of conventional dentistry for many people. Nor are words adequate to describe the satisfaction which so many patients feel following successful treatment by dental implants and restorative dentistry.

This book is also written for that which cannot be adequately conveyed in words.

Foreword

Osseointegrated reconstructions create a stomathognato–physiological situation which differs from that of the original dentate state.

Bone and marrow tissue, when used for anchorage of prosthetic devices according to the principles of osseointegration, provide a more rigid fixation than that of conventional crown and bridge work anchored to teeth, which are connected to the jaw bone via the resilient periodontium. This different biomechanical situation thus requires other technical considerations and procedures other than those developed for conventional intra–oral prostheses.

It is particularly important that the necessity of a team effort is recognised, and that the requirement of possible lifetime function of the prosthesis and the importance of a perfect passive fit are emphasised.

Meticulous precision in every detail in the creation of the prosthesis in the osseo-integrated superstructure is a decisive prerequisite for an adequate and lasting reconstruction.

This book contains the necessary information on technical procedures and on how to achieve a predictable prosthetic prognosis in clinical reality.

The Institute for Applied Biotechnology
Gothenburg, April, 1992
Professor P-I Brånemark MD, PhD, ODhc, MDhc, ScDhc.

Acknowledgements

My grateful thanks are due to those who helped with what is contained in this book. This took several forms. John Brooks, Director of Quintessence Publishing Company, UK, certainly deserves thanks for providing the original encouragement to write this book. I must also thank Precious Metal Techniques, London, who provided items for photography as did Nobelpharma AB, Gothenburg, Sweden, who also allowed me to copy items of their art work.

Colleagues Anthony Johnson and David Wildgoose generously allowed me to show examples of their work. Anthony in chapter 11, and David in chapters 4, 10 and 11. Barry Cayless—Smith of Regent Dental Limited, Leighton Buzzard, UK, contributed technical work to chapters 6, 10 and 11 and elsewhere. I am grateful to these artist—craftsmen. In the true spirit of learning I would also thank all those from this country and overseas who allowed me to see examples of less flattering technical and clinical work. We all have examples of this.

Mary Brook—Smith kindly allowed me to use parts of her University of Sheffield Mechanical Engineering final year research project and Professor David Newland and his staff in the Department of Mechanical Engineering at the University of Cambridge helped with the fatigue testing of frameworks and implant screws.

Particular thanks are due to Professor Richard Johns and Raymond Winstanley of the Sheffield School of Clinical Dentistry for such a multiplicity of things that it is impossible for me to even hint at them here.

It is a special pleasure to be able to thank Professor P-I Brånemark. He provided two gifts, a flattering foreword and the guiding notion that persistent precision provides predictable prognosis.

I reserve my greatest thanks for my wife Gillian, and sons Paul and Christopher. All that I have achieved has been with their help and without them none of this would have been possible.

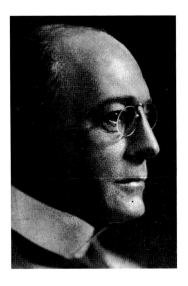

This book is
Dedicated to the Memory
of
William H Taggart DDS
1855–1933

Implant dental technology has at its centre the art and science of precision lost–wax casting. This technology, which is more than 4500 years old, was transformed as recently as 1907 when Chicago dentist William Taggart published his method of pressure casting gold rather than pouring it from a ladle. Taggart's profound contribution to dentistry and to the manufacturing industry has been inadequately recognised. We must all be grateful to him. This book is humbly dedicated to his memory.

Glossary of
Special Terms Used

Since the introduction of successful dental implants new dental terms have come into common usage which are not contained in the *Dental vocabulary Part 1. General and clinical terms*. (1). Additional to these are several terms developed by the author for use in dental technology. These are used in the text as follows:

Abutment cylinder
A trans–mucosal extension of a fixture which provides an intra–oral connection terminal.

Abutment replica
A copy of the titanium abutment cylinder which is attached to copings in impressions so that replicas occupy the same positions in casts as titanium abutments occupy in the mouth.

Abutment screw
A titantium or gold alloy bolt which joins the abutment cylinder to the fixture.

Compound prosthesis
A two-part construction consisting of an implant supported metal sub–frame and congruent separate prosthesis, the whole joined by screws.

Cantilever implant
One of a group of implants connected by a framework from which originates a cantilever.

Cantilever teeth
Posterior teeth which are entirely supported by a framework cantilever.

Casting-on
The process by which prefabricated metal components contained in a pattern are incorporated into a casting without soldering.

Crucible former
A cone–shaped device which makes a depression in an investment mould for the purpose of concentrating molten metal over sprue orifices.

Two-part dental implant
A bio–compatible bone anchor and connected abutment cylinder complete.

Fixed prosthesis
A prosthesis which is screw connected to its supporting implants and cannot be removed by the patient.

Fixture
A biocompatible bone anchor with a sub—gingival abutment connection terminal.

Fixture terminal
That part of a fixture to which a trans—mucosal abutment is connected.

Framework
A discrete accurately fitting metal beam contained within a prosthesis. Used to provide strength adequate to resist functional loads and transmit these loads to bone via the implants.

Gold cylinder
A Platinum alloy cylinder which forms the connection between a prosthesis and supporting implants.

When incorporated within a prosthesis it provides a fixed denture rational. When attached to implants external to the prosthesis it allows the retention of an overdenture.

Gold cylinder skirt
A smooth external margin of metal encircling a gold cylinder adjacent to its fitting surface.

Gold screw
Yellow gold alloy bolt used to clamp gold cylinders to either abutment replicas or implants.

Impression copings
Metal blocks which are attached to abutments in the mouth to form a registration of implant positions in impressions.

Implant number
A numbering system which identifies the position of an implant relative to a loaded cantilever. For example implant Number 1 is a cantilever implant, 2 the next implant removed from the cantilever, 3 the next and so on. Fig 5-1 illustrates the system.

Intermediate prosthesis
A prosthesis worn during prosthesis and/or bone tissue remodelling development.

Mature bone
Bone formed on and adjacent to osseointegrated fixtures which has undergone a remodelling adaptation to applied functional stress.

Novice bone
Newly healed bone formed on and adjacent to osseointegrated fixtures.

Novice cantilever length
An abbreviated cantilever which will eventually require extending to a final or mature length.

Novice occlusion
A temporary reduction of the number and/or size of artificial posterior teeth to provide a reduced occlusal table.

Novice prosthesis
A denture of final construction carrying fewer or narrower teeth to provide a reduced occlusal table. Denture worn during post—osseointegration bone re—modelling.

Osseointegration
A direct structural and functional connection between ordered living bone and the surface of an implanted fixture.

Osseo—disintegration

A prosthesis induced stress overload of osseointegrated implants, prosthetic components and/or supporting bone tissue resulting in their degeneration or failure.

Overdenture

A patient removable prosthesis which covers completely at least one implant and is retained by retentive connection to one or more implants.

Overdenture retainers

Type 1 Where resilient clips contained in a prosthesis grasp a bar joining two or more implants.

Type 2 Where individual connectors contained in a prosthesis separately connect with individual implants.

Pattern chamber

Cavity contained in an investment mould formed by the evacuation of a pattern during mould heating.

Reduced occlusal table

The provision of artificial teeth with narrower bucco—lingual and/or mesio—distal occlusal surface dimensions than the finally used artificial teeth.

Retrievability

The ease by which devices, components or prostheses may be recovered from the mouth.

Safe bearing

The margin of safety by which implants and their bone bed foundations can resist functional stress from a prosthesis.

Sheffield fit test

The fit applying between technical work and abutment replicas and/or implants when only one gold fixing screw is remotely tightened to place.

Slave gold screws

Gold screws for exclusive laboratory use.

Sleeping fixture

An osseointegrated fixture without connection to an abutment.

Sprue former

A wax rod.

Stent

A plate worn by a patient during fixture installation which indicates to the surgeon where individual fixtures should be placed.

Stock teeth

Commercially manufactured artificial teeth.

Temporary prosthesis

A modified existing denture worn during the period of fixture osseointegration and final prosthesis construction.

REFERENCE

1. BS EN 21942–1: 1992. (ISO 1942–1). *Dental vocabulary Part 1. General and clinical terms.* British Standards Institution, London.

Chapter One

Introduction

From the very beginning dentistry has attempted to devise an artificial replacement for the missing tooth and its root. The notion of implanting pins or other devices into the jaw to serve as denture stabilisers has long been theoretically attractive. But, despite many attempts and the use of promising materials as these became available, the number of implants which were secure in the mouth after 5 years was until recently unacceptably low.

This situation was completely reversed in 1981 when Professor P-I Brånemark and his co–workers published what has now become recognised as one of the most important scientific papers ever published in dentistry.[1] Brånemark demonstrated that he had developed the first reliable dental implant. Also evident was the fact that the implant and the protocol for its use were founded on meticulous scientific research, work which was combined with imaginative mechanical and metallurigical innovation (Fig 1-1).

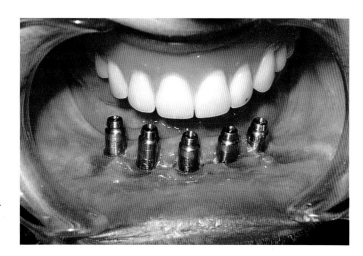

Fig 1-1 *Osseointegrated Brånemark dental implants installed in an edentulous mouth in order to support a complete prosthesis.*

THE BRÅNEMARK DENTAL IMPLANT

After his investigations into the micro–circulation of blood in the rabbit where he had inserted titanium observation chambers in the tibia, Brånemark found that he could not remove his devices. Living bone had joined with the surface of the inserted metal. Further investigation confirmed that commercially pure titanium, or more accurately its oxide coating, was reliably acceptable to human as well as rabbit bone.

The Brånemark implant comprises five parts, (Fig 1-2): a titanium fixture a), abutment cylinder b), abutment screw c), gold cylinder d) and gold screw e). The fixture, which is externally threaded for initial stability on insertion in bone, has a bone chip collector and chamber arranged at its apex a). The abutment, which forms the trans–mucosal component, is connected to the fixture by an abutment screw. To these surgically installed components is added a gold cylinder and its screw. Components which form a machined interface by which technical work is connected to bone via intermediary supporting implants (Fig 1-3, page 22).

Knowing the poor reputation of contemporary implants at that time Brånemark delayed a complete description of his methods until he could show long–term clinical evidence. His success has excited intensive alternative work elsewhere. As a prelude to the formation of an International Standard for Dental Implants, the International Organization for Standardization (ISO) has compiled a Technical Report which lists experimental and clinically available dental implants (ISO TR 10451).[2] From this it is evident that almost every conceivable implant design, material and combination of materials is now receiving attention.

The Brånemark implant was the first dental implant to receive an Acceptability recognition by the American Dental Association. This commendation relates to its use in the edentulous mouth, with other clinical uses obtaining Provisional Acceptance. Others, more prominently Core–vent and IMZ implants have Provisional Acceptance for use in the edentulous mouth. In the United Kingdom, the Department of Health National Health Service Procurement Directorate has approved the manufacture of Brånemark and Straumann dental implants in relation to their Good Manufacturing Guide.

There are now so many look–alike imitations of Brånemark and other successful implants that dentistry faces increasing difficulties of choice, specially in the face of claim and counter claim. This similarity, however, is advantageous in that the dental technology which is required for many implants is comparable, if not identical to that required by the Brånemark implant. Unnecessary repetition can, therefore, be usefully avoided by using the Brånemark implant as the reference implant system described in this text.

THE USE OF IMPLANTS

Implants may be used whatever the extent and pattern of tooth loss. A special indication, however, is in those mouths where an edentulous lower jaw has deteriorated from the time that the original dentures were fitted.

Typically, in these circumstances, conventional lower dentures are difficult if not impossible to wear because of instability and pain. The required implant supported

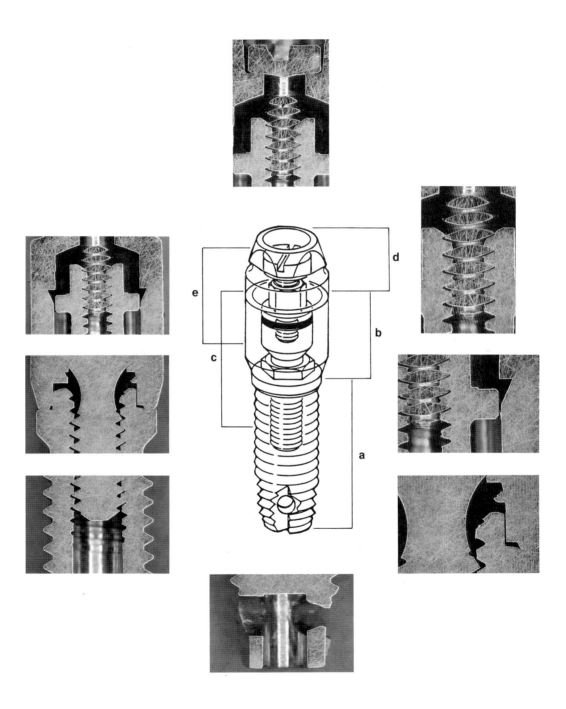

Fig 1-2 *The Brånemark dental implant showing its internal parts.*

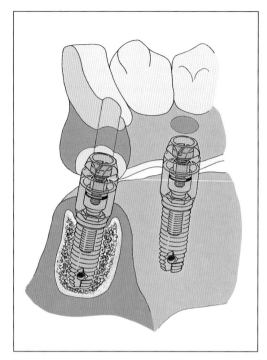

Fig 1-3 *Prosthesis screw connected to its implant and bone foundations.*

prosthesis may be fixed in the mouth or be patient removable. The former type is conventional in almost every respect, except that it contains within itself a partly concealed metal framework. This has the important function of passively connecting the exposed implant parts which protrude into the mouth. The framework must also be strong enough to withstand masticatory forces without fracture or permanent deformation and safely transmit these loads to its supporting implants and their bone bed. Such prostheses are screwed in place and cannot be removed by the patient (Fig 1-3).

In the early part of this century pioneer Alfred Gysi ingeniously explained how the occlusion of the teeth in complete den-

tures should be related to the temporomandibular joints and their envelope of movement. Using the analogy of gear wheels Gysi showed how alignment inaccuracies of the wheels would occasion gear teeth interferences, which in artificial teeth caused denture movement and pain (Fig 1-4 a). To the present day occlusal balance is assuredly useful only when the dentures are securely in place. Even in mouths where the residual ridges are highly resorbed, implant supported prostheses offer the reliable prospect of relating the occlusion of the teeth to the movements of the temporomandibular joints (Fig 1-4 b).

Brånemark called the necessary bone—to—implant union 'osseointegration'. The long—term preservation of osseointegration has been shown to depend to a considerable extent on the prosthesis having a passive connection to its supporting implants. A passive fitting is characterized by a complete absence of rocking or vertical and horizontal misfitting gaps without fixing screws or alternatively the fit obtaining when only one fixing screw is remotely tightened to place. (See Glossary, Sheffield fit test). A passive fit and 'fitting without gaps' are quite different and should not be confused. A correct tightening in place of a distorted framework in the mouth has the effect of closing misfitting gaps to give the appearance of a satisfactory fit. This is dangerously deceptive. Continuous compressive, tensile and/or bending forces will be resolved in the implants. Depending on their magnitude, such loads can be destructive both to the implant and its host bone. To these potentially serious problems must be added the inconvenience to the patient if the prosthesis, framework or implant parts break. Apart form the difficult repair that may be necessary, the pa-

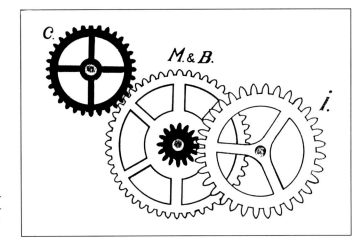

Fig 1-4 a *Gysi's representation of the dynamic interdependence of the temporomandibular joints (C), molars and premolars (M & B) and incisors (i) if occlusal balance is to be obtained. A theorem which is spoiled by denture instability.*

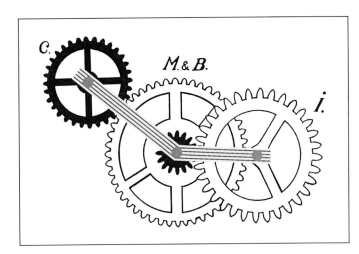

Fig 1-4 b *When artificial teeth are joined to the jaws by implants, their occlusal surfaces can then be accurately integrated with each other and with the temporomandibular joints.*

tient may swallow or inhale the broken parts.

Flushed with the success of osseointegration, reviewers and researchers alike have placed the very highest credence on the statistical success rates of individual implants measured after healing and at yearly intervals thereafter. This work is usually unhelpful, if not misleading. Although the survival rate of implants is closely related to their ability to bear functional loads, accounts of longevity rarely, if ever, include details of the load stress to which both surviving and failed implants have been subjected.[1-10] This is an important omission.

Such reports come from established teams and researchers from teaching institutions with extensive experience. New teams will have to ascend a learning curve based on their own experiences. Until more data is available, prosthesis design must be undertaken cautiously, with implant and bone preservation overwhelmingly in mind.

Brånemarks' great contribution has been to demonstrate how osseointegration may be reliably obtained, provided that a specific clinical protocol is followed. To this success must be added the need for a similarly prescribed dental technology if osseointegration is to be preserved long—term. Paradoxically, current implant dental technology occupies the same position as implants themselves had before the definitive work of Brånemark became widely accepted. Implant dental technology is largely anecdotal and is practised as a subject of trial and error.

SHEFFIELD DENTAL TECHNOLOGY AND RESEARCH

Much of the technology described in these pages has been developed by the author in the University of Sheffield School of Clinical Dentistry and used there in the treatment of patients since 1985. Arising from this, a 'Sheffield Method' of implant dental technology is now practiced in several University Dental Schools, commercial dental laboratories and Military Establishments in the United Kingdom and elsewhere.

The objective of this method is to provide a dental technology as reliably predictable as the Brånemark implant to which it is connected. Centrally important a method of routinely casting one—piece, lightweight, and clinically unbreakable frameworks has been developed which does not require corrective soldering. Not only is this structure a reliably passive fit, but substantial savings in production costs have been made over alternative methods of fabrication. No part of the method or materials used for making frameworks has changed since 1985.

The research and practical details of framework design and construction described in Chapters 5 and 7 were recognised by the City and Guilds of London Institute who awarded their 1989 Gold Medal for Innovation and Excellence in Craftsmanship.

OSSEOINTEGRATED IMPLANTS

In predicting future trends in international dental health care, it has been asserted that dental implants will be increasingly used to replace single teeth or entire dental arches as an alternative to dentures and other restorative work.[11] It is hoped that this prediction is incorrect. Patients certainly do not want dental implants. That these devices may carry a high probability of achieving a direct and satisfactory union with living bone is not sufficient reason for their use.

Implants are unattractive in appearance, inefficient for mastication and do little to aid speech (Fig 1-1). This, however, is not their function. Implants are foundations, albeit radical ones, for future prosthetic therapy. What is attractive to patients is the promise of a securely stable, retentive and enduring prosthesis of minimal bulk. Reason enough when the mouth provides poor or difficult foundations for conventional dentures.

OSSEO—DISINTEGRATION

Osseointegrated implants are not inviolate. There have been many reports of broken implant parts and framework cantilevers, fixture loss, loosening of the prosthesis in function and accelerated bone loss.[1,5,7,12,13,14] All are avoidable treatment complications which conspire to undermine dental implants as the basis of a reliable treatment option. Many failures can be traced to an inadequate dental technology which acts to spoil what careful fixture installation, successful healing and patient co-operation have established. Even when implant and bone loss problems do not occur, an unreliable prosthesis carries with it the patients opinion of implant failure as a treatment option. It is of lesser importance to the returning patient that the implants may still be securely in place.

Informed technical work, by contrast, reduces the likelihood of failure of implants and bone by increasing the margins of functional safety of prostheses. This is especially so in mouths where short or malplaced implants have been installed and where poor bone conditions exist.

that the sometimes separate disciplines of prosthetic and conservative technology are combined.

Most conservative dental technology is provided for medium to long–term treatment and all conventional prosthetic care relatively short term. Osseointegrated implants offer a routine treatment modality with the unprecedented promise of lasting the patient's life-time. Dentistry has yet to recognise the implications of this and the continuing prosthesis maintenance and other patient support which will be increasingly necessary in the future. Long-term treatment planning can involve difficult decisions of prosthesis design. For example, that which may be presently provided with reduced cleaning access for reasons of appearance, may be inappropriate in later years. Age, and possible infirmity may then conspire to reduce a patient's ability to maintain necessary oral hygiene procedures and to obtain professional help.

TEAM–WORK

Successfull treatment depends not only on the active co-operation of the patient, but also on the co-operation of the entire implant team before, during and after implant installation. Even when the laboratory is unavoidably distant from clinical activity, the technician must not be. An ethic so often thought to be desirable elsewhere in dentistry, is essential here. Above all, the usually separate disciplines of dental technology, prosthodontics and oral surgery must be intimately co-ordinated. A similar rationalisation must also occur within dental technology itself, so

TRAINING

At present only a very few research based courses on implant dental technology are available for technicians. The best of the more usual courses is where the entire team are trained together, with each member being made aware of the responsibilities and duties of the others. Training and follow–up support is as crucially necessary for dental technology as it is for the clinical aspects of implant work. Although some implant manufacturers may choose to provide clinical advisory staff, fewer provide any authoritative technical expertise.

PERSISTENT PRECISION PROVIDES PREDICTABLE PROGNOSIS

Osseointegrated implants bring with them the ability to integrate the teeth with the jaws and the temporomandibular joints. The occlusion of the teeth can now be that which is clinically necessary and not that which is dictated by unstable dentures. Prostheses which are fixed in place in the mouth are entirely stable in function with the ability to bite and chew food restored to the former dentate state.

A successful implant supported prosthesis restores more than the teeth. Denture problems often give rise to personal and social impairments of deep and un—admitted importance. These too can be restored by a successful prosthesis. By the use of secure implant foundations a more complete patient care is possible and fundamental to these exciting possibilities is the quality of dental technology support provided. Technology has the responsibility of providing technical work which will durably compliment the success of osseointegrated implants of whatever manufacture. Dental technology certainly has the ability to undermine if not deny that which otherwise can be so confidently promised.

REFERENCES

1. Adell R, Leckholm U, Rockler B, Brånemark, P-I: A 15-year study of osseointegrated implants in the treatment of the edentulous jaw. *Int J Oral Surg* 1981; 10: 387–416.

2. ISO TR 10451. Dental implants—State of the art—Survey of materials. First edition 1991. International Organization for Standardization, Geneva, Switzerland.

3. Albrektsson T, Zarb G, Worthington P, Eriksson A R. The long-term efficacy of currently used dental implants: A review and proposed criteria of success: *Int J Oral & Maxillofac Implants* 1986; 1: 11–25.

4. Steenberghe van D, Quirynen M, Calberson L, Demanet M. A prospective evaluation of the fate of 697 consecutive intra—oral fixtures modum Brånemark in the rehabilitation of edentulism. *J Head & Neck Pathol* 1987; 6: 53–57.

5. Cox J F, Zarb G. The longitudinal clinical efficacy of osseointegrated dental implants: A 3—year report. *Int J Oral & Maxillofac Implants* 1987; 2: 91–100.

6. Engquist B, Bergendal T, Kallus T, Linden U. A retrospective multicenter evaluation of osseointegrated implants supporting overdentures. *Int J Oral & Maxillofac Implants* 1988; 3: 129–134.

7. Albrektsson T. A multicenter report on osseointegrated oral implants. *J Prosth Dent* 1988; 60: 75–84.

8. Albrektsson T, Zarb G. The Brånemark Osseointegrated Implant 1989: 229–232. Quintessence Publishing Co, Inc Chicago, USA.

9. Ahlqvist J, Borg K, Gunne J, Nilson H, Olsson M, Astrand P. Osseointegrated implants in edentulous jaws: A 2—year longitudinal study. *Int J Oral & Maxillofac Implants* 1990; 5: 155–163.

10. Jemt T. Failures and complications in 391 consecutively inserted fixed prostheses supported by Brånemark implants in edentulous jaws: A study of treatment from the time of prosthesis placement to the first annual checkup. *Int J Oral & Maxillofac Implants* 1991; 6: 270–275.

11. Simonsen R J. Dentistry in the 21st Century: A global perspective. Proceedings of the International Symposium on Dentistry in the 21st Century, Berlin, September 10, 1989. 1991; Quintessence Publishing Co, Inc Berlin, Germany.

12. Gregory M, Murphy W M, Scott J, Watson C J, Reeve P E. A clinical study of the Brånemark dental implant system. *Brit Dent J* 1990; 168: 18–23.

13. Lindquist L W, Carlsson G E, Glantz P-O. Rehabilitation of the edentulous mandible with tissue integrated fixed prosthesis: A six year longitudinal study. *Quintessence Int* 1987; 12: 11–16.

14. Johansson G, Palmqvist S. Complications, supplementary treatment, and maintenance in edentulous arches with implant—supported fixed prostheses: *Int J Pros* 1990; 3: 89–92.

Chapter Two
Laboratory equipment

Laboratories need to be furnished with equipment for full denture construction and crown and bridge—work, other than this no other special apparatus is required. A timed vacuum investing machine is essential, with a selection of larger sizes of mixing vessels (Fig 2-1 a). A great assistance in the cleaning of prosthodontic kit and implant parts, and particularly the fitting surfaces of castings and abutment replicas, is the pressure steam cleaner. Safer than its name suggests the pressure steam cleaner can efficiently remove wax, polishing compounds and other debris from even the most inaccessible crevices (Fig 2-1 b) (a). Equally useful is the compressed air powered, glass bead polishing — aluminium oxide particle abrading cabinet; metal surface cleaning and its preparation for other processes is greatly facilitated by this simple apparatus.

If pre—weighed packets of investment powder are not used, then accurate electric weighing scales are essential in order to weigh investment powders from bulk.

Fig 2-1 a *Vacuum investing machine with built-in mixing timer and vibrator.*

Fig 2-1 b *Pressure steam cleaner.*

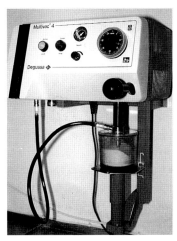

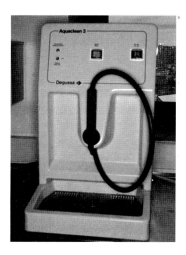

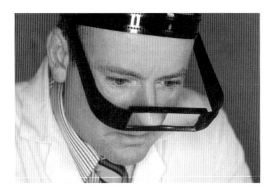

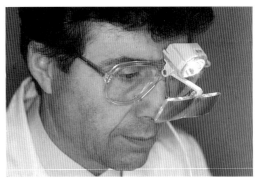

Fig 2-2 a (above left) *Convenient and inexpensive head band loupe.*

Fig 2-2 b (above right) *Individual lens magnifiers with central light.*

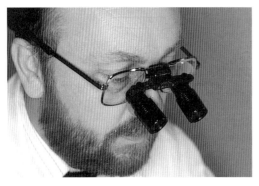

Fig 2-2 c *Prismatic eye telescopes fitted to special spectacle frames.*

Some additional smaller items are also useful. Implants and prosthetic kit consist of parts which are small and easily lost. Gold screws are particularly diminutive, with threads that are easily damaged by mishandling.

Suitably small screwdrivers are available for a wide variety of home workshop uses. Avoid these in favour of those supplied by the implant manufacturer. Correctly fitting screwdriver blades are essential if gold screw head damage is to be avoided. Even with this precaution it is good practice to retain a set of slave screws for exclusive laboratory use.

Plastic work boxes which contain individual loose boxes, or single compartmentalised boxes are useful to store and identify components during technical

work. Prosthetic kit such as impression copings, guide pins, gold screws and other parts are delivered with technical work for individual patients. These components will need to be identified and separated from other material before returning as appropriate. Small tweezers with well fitting beaks are indispensable for handling these small parts.

A storage and index system also proves useful for the stock of implant and prosthodontic parts kept in the laboratory.

MAGNIFICATION

The required technology necessitates attention to detail; work which is easier when eye magnification is used. For general work, a X4 magnification head band loupe is inexpensive and very useful (b). However the type MXL Voroscope is more effective with individual lens magnifiers attached to spectacle frames incorporating a convenient light (c). Prismatic eye telescopes provide the best quality magnification.

A times 3 magnification array with 340 mm working distance and 62 mm field of view is convenient and not especially heavy (d) (Figs 2-2 a–c). All three types may be raised for direct vision.

A searching and final arbiter of excellence is the illuminating stereoscopic microscope of X20 magnification. No dental laboratory should be without this indispensable aid to quality control.

CHAPTER 2: MATERIALS AND EQUIPMENT

Manufacturer

UK Suppliers

(a) Multivac 4
Aquaclean 3
Degussa AG
Postfach 110533
D-6000 Frankfurt
Germany

Degussa Limited
Winterton House
Winterton Way
Macclesfield
SK11 0LP

(b) Lactona x4 head band loupe
Lactona
Brouwerijbaan 8–12
PO Box 326
4600 AH Bergen
Op-Zoom, Holland

Precious Metal Techniques
29 Chiltern Street
London
W1M 1 HG

(c) Voroscope loupe type MXL
Australian Biomedical Corp Ltd
39 DeHavilland Road
Mordialloc
Victora 3195
Australia

Garth Jessamine Health Care
PO Box 108
Wokingham
RG11 2 GU

(d) Prismatic eye telescopes
Keeler Limited
Clewer Hill Road
Windsor
SL4 4AA

Chapter Three
The Installation of Implants

A radiographic examination of the patients jaws determines the architecture of the bone and the position of the mental nerve in the mandible. Fixtures are installed with regard to both features and to the position of natural teeth.

Brånemark discovered that successful osseointegration was more likely when newly installed fixtures were not loaded during the period of bone healing. For this reason he concluded that the implant must be used in two parts. First, the fixture is installed so that it is contained and protected within bone. Only after confirmed osseointegration is the abutment or second implant part screw connected to the fixture. Thus the two—part Brånemark implant requires a two stage surgical operation; events which are separated by the necessary interval in which to achieve a bone to fixture union. Except for certain implants for exclusive single tooth use, most successful implants have a two—part construction and installation.

Before beginning work teams will find it advantageous to have a clearly delineated treatment plan. With this in mind, primary impressions and provisional jaw registration will allow study casts to be mounted onto an articulator in preparation for the next stage which is pre-surgical treatment planning. This is one of the most important stages in the prevention of future prosthetic/technological difficulties, if not treatment failure.

Pre—surgical treatment planning

A group comprising the technician, prosthodontist and oral surgeon will consider the patients needs with regard to the:
- number and position of required fixtures.
- maximum height of abutments with regard to available space, including occlusal plane height limitations.
- minimum height of abutments bearing in mind an easy cleaning access of the abutments and under parts of the prosthesis.
- use of special abutments for the partially dentate or where abutment concealment is necessary.

When unhelpful jaw relationships and/or natural teeth are present, other conditions apply. There is a possibility that the primary models may need to be mounted onto an adjustable articulator to determine possible tooth interferences with implants and framework parts. In difficult cases it is helpful when a tentative tooth set—up is made. This enables the most effective positions for fixtures to be assessed and marked on the casts for use by the surgeon.

When more experience has been gained, collective discussions of this

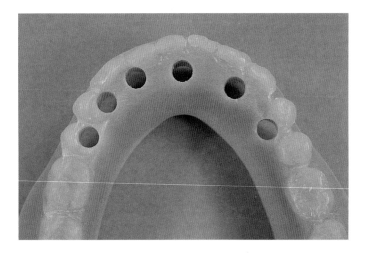

Fig 3-1 a *Duplicate complete denture with holes indicating implant positions.*

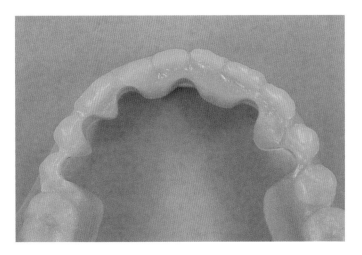

Fig 3-1 b *Lingual denture parts cut away to provide drill access guides.*

depth may only be required for more difficult mouths, especially those that are partially dentate.

A variety of problems, including some severe technical ones can be caused by the malplaced implant. Experienced surgeons have few problems of this sort and even these can be reduced by the use of surgical drilling stents.

DRILLING STENTS

In their simplest form drilling stents are made by providing drill access holes and alignment guides in an autopolymerised resin duplicate of the patients existing denture (Figs 3-1a and b). This type of stent has the advantage of indicating the required implant position and alignment in relation to the opposing jaw. As the number of required prosthetic teeth diminishes so the position of implants becomes

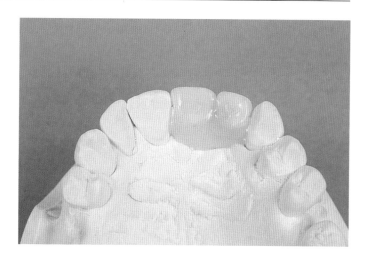

Fig 3-2 a *Resin teeth positioned to restore appearance.*

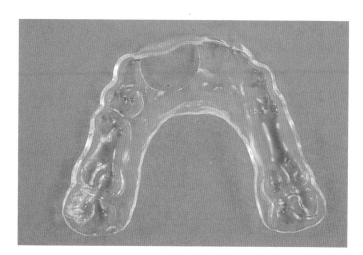

Fig 3-2 b *Vacuum formed stent trimmed and polished showing its fitting surface.*

more critically prescribed. With the single tooth or small prosthesis in the front of the mouth the use of a drilling stent is mandatory, even for experienced teams.

A plate resembling a bite raising appliance makes a useful stent. Having first set correctly sized resin stock teeth in a study cast (Fig 3-2 a), a 1.5 mm thick sheet of Biocryl material (a) is vacuum adapted overall. The material covers the occlusal and palatal tooth surfaces and extends approximately 2 mm onto the labial and buccal tooth surfaces to provide retention. After trimming and smoothing, the plate covering the palatal surfaces of the replacement teeth is ground away to provide drill access to the fixture sites. Only a labial shell covering of the replacement teeth remains (Figs 3-2 b–d). The surgeon can now arrange drilling instruments with regard to the positions of the fixtures, artificial teeth and access holes of the screws used to retain the prosthesis.

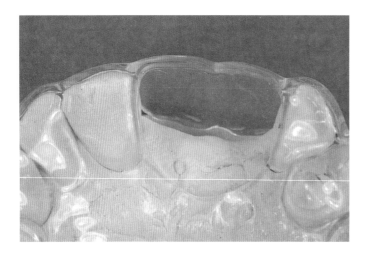

Fig 3-2 c   *Plate ground away to provide access to fixture installation sites.*

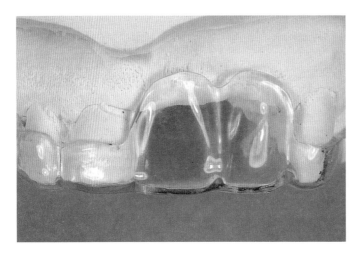

Fig 3-2 d   *Tooth shell representations of the future prosthetic teeth. Note plate extension onto the teeth to provide retention.*

Because the stent is formed on the outside of the cast, the labial surfaces of the stent teeth are 1.5 mm anterior to the future replacement teeth. The surgeon must compensate for this when deciding on the anterior/posterior position of the fixtures.

This difficulty can be avoided when a plate carrying resin artificial teeth in their correct position is used. A provided drill access aperture is then enlarged in an anterior direction until only the thinnest labial veneers of the original teeth remain (Figs 3-3 a and b). These tooth surfaces are positioned accurately to enable the surgeon to place fixtures in precise relation to the future replacement teeth (Fig 3-3 c).

Dental appearance, abutment cleaning access, gold and implant screw longevity, prosthesis size and shape and the ease by which good technical work can be carried out is largely decided by the fixture position.

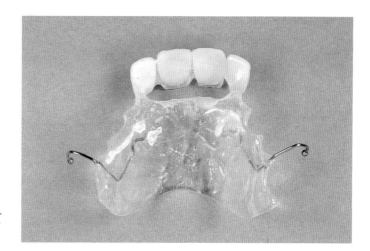

Fig 3-3 a *Drilling stent consisting of resin stock teeth, clear base and wire retainers.*

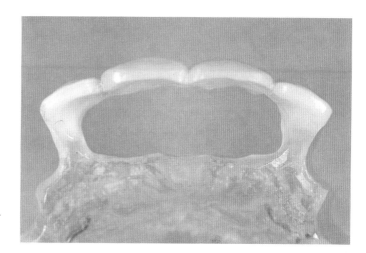

Fig 3-3 b *Plate and tooth material ground away to provide thin labial tooth shells.*

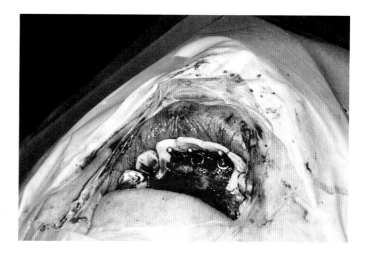

Fig 3-3 c *Stent in use. Note fixture positions close up to the tooth shells.*

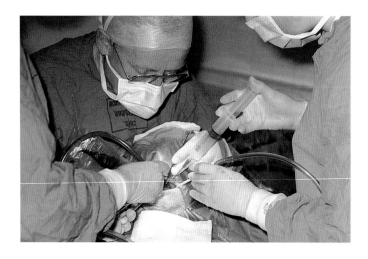

Fig 3-4 a *The surgical installation of fixtures is a closely co-ordinated team effort.*

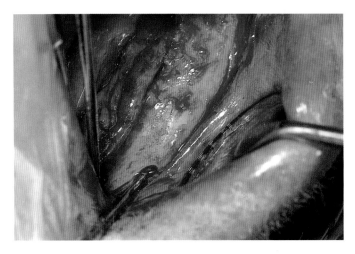

Fig 3-4 b *Mandibular bone exposed from soft tissues.*

FIXTURE INSTALLATION

In edentulous jaws the minimum number of fixtures necessary to support a fixed prosthesis is four and two fixtures are minimally required for a removable overdenture. Surgical installation is usually done in one visit, with the patient under sedation and either local or general anaesthesia.

Sometimes four or more fixtures will be installed, but only two used to support a transitional overdenture. At a later stage the sleeping fixtures will be activated and a fixed prosthesis made. Prostheses for the partially dentate require as many fixtures as can be conveniently installed without crowding.

The implant installation sites are exposed from soft tissue and using drills of increasing diameter, holes are prepared in the bone followed by countersinking and threading. The surgeon places fixtures of sufficient length in order to en-

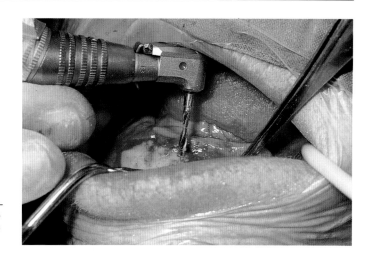

Fig 3-4 c *Twist drills of increasing size are used to prepare holes of the correct diameter to receive fixtures.*

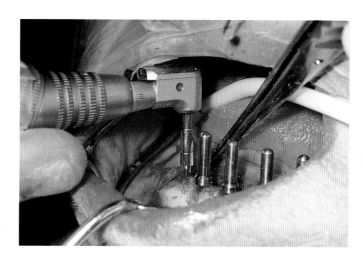

Fig 3-4 d *Direction indicator pins help the surgeon with parallel drilling.*

gage the maximum depth of available bone (Figs 3-4 a–d). Brånemark found that a reduction of frictional heat generated during drilling was essential to successful bone healing. For this reason carefully controlled drilling speeds and profuse saline spray drill cooling are used (Figs 3-5 a and b). The fixtures are placed approximately 3.5 to 4 mm apart, giving a centre to centre implant distance of 7 to 8 mm.

In inexperienced hands angulated abutments (Chapter 6) are used as a contingency procedure to alter difficult implant positions, as these are discovered immediately prior to or during prosthetic care. Practised surgeons can cleverly minimise such difficulties at the time of fixture installation by anticipating the future use of angulated abutments when they deliberately choose to install accurately tilted bone finding fixtures.

When fixtures have been installed, protective metal caps are screw connected to the exposed terminals of the fixtures, a

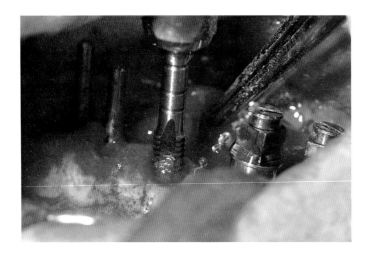

Fig 3-5 a *Prepared hole being threaded under saline spray cooling.*

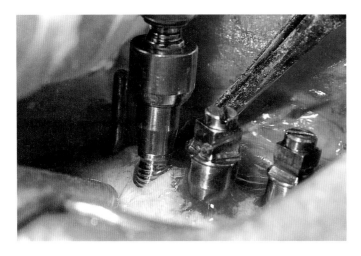

Fig 3-5 b *Installation of a Bråne-mark fixture under spray cooled conditions.*

precaution which prevents bone forming in their internal threaded parts. Returned sutured soft tissue is then positioned to completely cover the installed fixtures. After this has healed the presence of the fixtures is not discernible, either to the patient or to the observer (Figs 3-5 c and d).

TEMPORARY PROSTHESES

Since osseointegration is less certain when fixtures are loaded before bone healing has taken place, some patients are not allowed to wear their existing dentures during this phase of treatment. Fortunately, this is not usually the case. Edentulous patients are pleased to have their dentures modified at the chairside with a temporary soft lining which is sufficiently extended in order to cover the buried fixtures. The provision of efficient temporary or provisional prostheses has important clinical as well as obvious social advan-

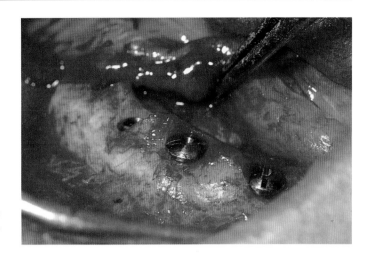

Fig 3-5 c *Cover screw attached to fixture terminal prior to the return of the soft tissues.*

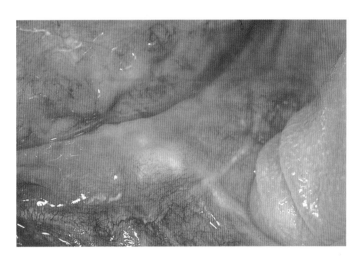

Fig 3-5 d *Appearance of healed mucosa. The presence of an implant can sometimes be detected by pressure from a finger tip which leaves a lighter area.*

tages for the patient. These are discussed in Chapter 4.

There then follows a period of clinical inactivity during which time new bone forms onto the acquiescent fixtures. This interval will occupy at least 3 months for mandibular fixtures, and between 4 and 5 months for maxillary fixtures. The extended maxillary healing time is necessary due to the poorer quality of bone usually found in this jaw. Surgeons will not hesitate to extend healing intervals if this is required.

ABUTMENT CONNECTION

Following uneventful healing, the patient returns to the operating chair for a second and simpler surgical procedure of abutment connection. A circular punch instrument removes soft tissue to expose the cover screws, the removal of which reveals the hexagonal heads of the fixture terminals. Shown here are two implants for an overdenture (Figs 3-6 a–d). Titanium abutment cylinders are then screw

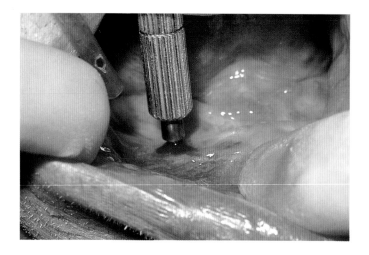

Fig 3-6 a *Soft tissue removal immediately over the fixture using a circular punch blade cutter.*

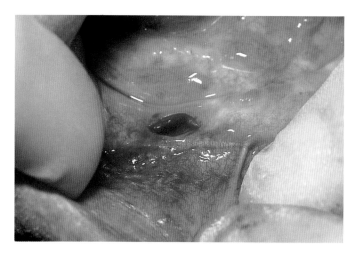

Fig 3-6 b *Removed tissue providing access to the cover screw.*

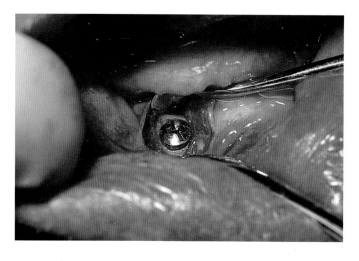

Fig 3-6 c *Exposed cover screw.*

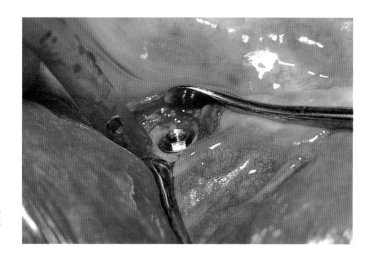

Fig 3-6 d *Exposed hexagonal terminal of the osseointegrated fixture.*

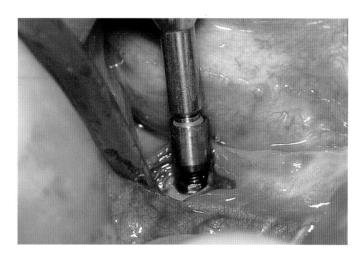

Fig 3-7 a *Connection of titanium abutment cylinder to the fixture.*

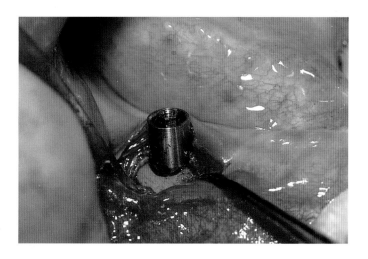

Fig 3-7 b *Installed abutment cylinder.*

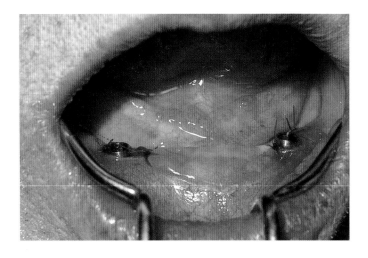

Fig 3-7 c   *Sutured soft tissues.*

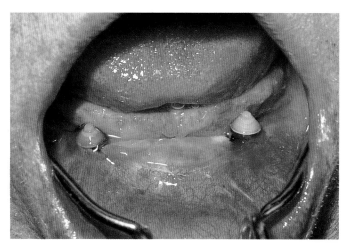

Fig 3-7 d   *Attached polymeric healing caps with lateral flanges to retain surgical pack.*

connected to these terminals. As a result of this connection a trans–mucosal implant terminal is then provided in the oral cavity (Figs 3-7 a and b). When the connected abutment is percussed with a metal instrument, successful osseointegration is indicated by a characteristic metallic ringing sound. It is the connection of the abutment cylinder to the fixture which essentially forms the implant (Fig 3-7 c).

Plastic healing caps are attached to abutments, protecting their machined fit-ting surfaces from damage and the ingress of debris. Two types are used in succession. The first has a lateral flange which is designed to retain surgical pack onto mucosal sutures (Fig 3-7 d). The second, which has approximately the same diameter as the abutment, is used after soft tissue healing (Fig 7-1 a). A soft lined denture may be worn over the smaller cap and its abutment during the period of prosthetic treatment which then follows.

42

Fig 3-8 a (left) *Bending moment obtaining when implants are arranged in a straight line.*

Fig 3-8 b (right) *Bending moment when implants are displaced relative to the occlusal surfaces of prosthetic teeth. a) is the point of application of occlusal force, b) the fulcrum and c) the resolved tension acting on the gold screw (Rangert et al.).*[1]

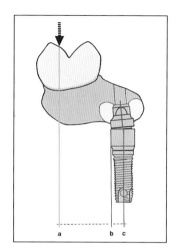

Because of its clearance from soft tissues, the construction of fixed prostheses may begin before complete mucosal healing has taken place. Patients often ask for this to be carried out, which is understandable. They are usually in a high state of expectation by this time. Because overdentures rest on mucosal tissue, patients requiring this treatment will have to wait for complete soft tissue healing before second impressions can be taken. The partially dentate will progress with further treatment depending on clinical circumstances.

IMPLANT POSITIONS

In avoiding the mental nerve, implants in the edentulous mandible will be grouped towards the anterior part of the jaw. Without such restrictions in the maxilla, implants in the upper jaw will be sited wherever the best bone is found and wherever the treatment plan allows. Consequently, maxillary implants may occupy more scattered positions.

It has been shown that in the edentulous jaw implants installed in a straight line are less able to tolerate cantilever loads than those arranged on a curve (Fig 3-8 a).[1] This is due to an opening effect on the screw joints from cantilever loads during function, with the consequence of adversely stressing the implant's gold and titanium connecting screws. Shortened cantilevers (Chapter 7), reduced occlusal tables and canine/premolar substitution will need to be used in these difficult circumstances (Chapter 8).

Masticatory forces applied to implants in a displaced position relative to the occlusal surfaces of artificial teeth also act to open screw joints and adversely stress implant screws (Fig 3-8 b).[1] Alternatively, when loads fall on implants more centrally situated under teeth, these are safely transmitted to bone along the long axis of the implant. Special technical difficulties are caused by an implant which is in an appropriate position but with an angulation which brings the gold screw access holes in the prosthesis into a conspicuous position. In extreme cases it is possible for angles to be formed between implants which will not allow the connection of a prosthesis.

Impossibly difficult technical problems may arise when these problems are combined. Angulated abutments will be immediately thought of, Chapter 6, but despite these and whatever technical ingenuity can be deployed, prosthesis connection difficulties, poor aesthetics, visible gold screw access holes, prosthesis overhang and unwelcome bulk can still remain.

FAILURE OF FIXTURES TO OSSEOINTEGRATE

Despite fixture loss during healing a change to the treatment plan may not be required. If five or six fixtures have been placed in an edentulous jaw the loss of one may not substantially alter the future prosthesis. An exception is when a cantilever fixture has been lost. In this case a framework with a longer cantilever than that desirably intended may be indicated.

Other difficulties arise when fixture loss places the treatment plan between one treatment option and another. For example, the intention to place a fixed prosthesis may necessitate revision in favour of a removable overdenture. Fortunately, this need only be a temporary recourse. Following the removal of the failed fixture and bone healing, another fixture can be installed into the same or an adjacent site and the original treatment plan resumed after this has osseointegrated.

A potentially more serious problem can arise when a fixture is lost in the partially dentate mouth. A single loss here can mean abandoning the original treatment plan until a replacement fixture has healed. Conventional adhesive bridges and removable partial dentures are conveniently available for the occasionally difficult intervening period.

THE TECHNICAL SIGNIFICANCE OF FIXTURE LOSS REPLACEMENT

When a new fixture is contained within the boundaries of an existing group of implants, the newly osseointegrated fixture will be supported by novice bone whereas elsewhere established implants and mature bone exist. With the advantage of this surrounding mature support no special consideration need be given to the new implant.

Alternatively, if the replacement fixture forms a new cantilever implant, its novice bone may require some load relief protection during its first year of post osseointegration bone maturation. A variety of methods are available to encourage this implant (Chapters 4 and 8).

REFERENCE

1. Rangert B, Jemt T, Jorneus L. Mechanical loading on Brånemark Implants. *Int J Oral & Maxillofac Implants* 1989; 4: 241–247.

CHAPTER 3: MATERIALS AND EQUIPMENT

Manufacturer	*UK Suppliers*
(a) Biocryl	
Scheu-Dental	Wright Health
D-5860 Iserlohn	Group Limited
Germany	Kingsway West
	Dundee
	DD2 3QD

Chapter Four
Provisional Prostheses

Depending on clinical needs provisional prostheses may be either temporary, intermediate or novice as follows:

- **Temporary prostheses.** A new or modified existing denture worn during the periods of fixture osseointegration healing, abutment connection and final prosthesis construction.
- **Intermediate prostheses.** A prosthesis worn after or instead of a temporary denture and designed specifically for the development of abutment cleaning access, appearance and occlusion of the teeth, and post–osseointegration bone remodelling.
- **Novice prostheses.** A denture of final construction but carrying fewer or narrower cantilever teeth used during the period of post–osseointegration bone remodelling.

TEMPORARY PROSTHESES

The wearing of soft lined existing dentures during the bone healing processes of fixture osseointegration has already been mentioned in Chapter 3. Through the use of these dentures the patient is in continual use of a prosthesis, except for the brief period of soft tissue healing when dentures cannot be worn at all.

Temporary dentures are always unsuitable in the sense that any existing deficiencies remain uncorrected and they cannot have a form or function which provides an introduction to the wearing of an implant supported prosthesis.

The interval between abutment connection and the delivery of the final prosthesis can be a trying time for the patient. Although surgery has been completed, protruding abutments now prevent the wearing of an existing prosthesis/restoration. Complete dentures can usually be modified again at the chairside by further alteration to their already ground fitting surfaces and provided temporary soft lining. With most metal partial dentures this is more complicated. Metalwork usually prevents the removal of sufficient denture base to accommodate abutments, making extensive grinding and/or denture extensions necessary; work which is often technically unsound and clinically unsatisfactory.

Correctly positioned fixtures and Cera-One and EsthetiCone abutments will prevent the wearing of existing temporary bridges. Sometimes, temporary bridges are designed to be capable of sufficient pontic modification to accomodate protruding abutments. If this has not been possible or the arrived positions of abutments preclude such revisions, a second temporary prosthesis will be necessary.

INTERMEDIATE PROSTHESES

Intermediate prostheses are worn for longer periods than is minimally necessary for the manufacture of the final prosthesis. Depending on circumstances, their size and shape can more closely approximate those of the final prosthesis, an advantage which offers an increased opportunity for prosthesis development. The shape, colour and position of teeth, their occlusion and overall prosthesis size are more easily evolved, with the patient becoming more accustomed to implant support. The effectiveness of a patients oral hygiene can also be monitored and cleaning access modifications to the prosthesis made if difficulties are found. Also valuable is the management of phonetic problems related to prosthesis to mucosa gaps occuring in the front of the mouth, which can be troublesome in maxillary prostheses.

Some time after fixture installation, healing, and subsequent prosthesis insertion, the bone reaches a 'steady state' of equilibrium.[1] The remodelling accommodation which occurs is the bone's constructive response to tolerable stress from the prosthesis via the implants. If by contrast, the applied stress exceeds that which is tolerable, the bone is absorbed. The reaction depends entirely on the magnitude and the frequency of the stress.

Intermediate prostheses can have the important additional role of assisting in the formation of reorganised mature bone by a more gradual functional loading of these tissues.[2] Not every patient will need this particular care. When, there are short fixtures and poor or grafted bone conditions, the more gradual loading provided by intermediate prostheses may be crucial to the preservation of osseointegration. Bone which has been functionally conditioned in this way will be more able to tolerate functional loads from mature final prostheses where otherwise, novice prostheses would need to be made. Intermediate prostheses are also used in mouths awaiting replacement implants when fixtures have been lost.

NOVICE PROSTHESES

This is where the final framework and tooth appearance have been furnished, but the cantilever teeth have reduced dimensions. Novice prostheses may be required in cases where implant and bone foundations are less well provided, this temporary recourse duplicates the function of intermediate prostheses in reducing the functional stress falling on these parts. The procedure is one of tooth narrowing and/or shortening during setting–up. Consequently, the subject is dealt with in Chapter 8. After a safe interval the prosthesis is altered by tooth additions, to provide an occlusal table of final dimensions.

THE CONSTRUCTION OF TEMPORARY AND INTERMEDIATE PROSTHESES

The single tooth

Despite an apparent lack of chemical bond with acrylic resin,[3] a successful resin temporary crown for the single incisor and CeraOne abutment may be made using a CeraOne plastic healing cap as its basis (Fig 4-1a).[4]

SR–Ivocron–PE crown and bridge resin is capable of providing a sufficiently adequate bond with a cap of reduced and

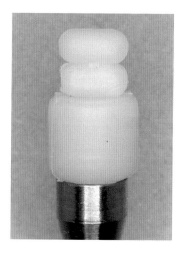

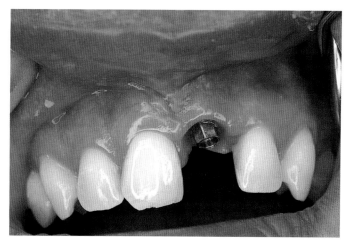

Fig 4-1 a (above, left) *Type DCA 126 plastic healing cap fitted on a CeraOne single tooth abutment.*

Fig 4-1 b (above right) *Installed CeraOne abutment. Note the already 'pre—formed' shape of the surrounding soft tissues.*

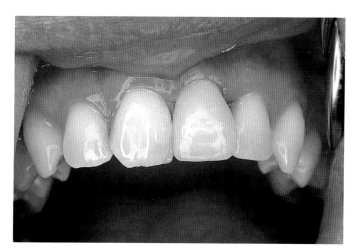

Fig 4-1 c *Completed temporary resin crown cemented to place.*

roughened surface, and a good appearance (Figs 4-1 b and c) (a).

Sheffield clips

Only intended to be used for a maximum of one year, these retainers are used in overdentures for mouths awaiting replacement implants. Made from round 1 mm diameter platinised wire, the clip essentially forms a clasp which engages an encircling groove contained in the older, but still available Nobelpharma gold cylinder type DCA 013 (Figs 4-2 a and b). Contemporary cylinders are less effective in that the necessary groove now has 4 intruding flat areas. Similar results can also be obtained using Temporary Retention Cylinders (Fig 4-2 c) (b). Intended for use under soft lined temporary dentures, these cylinders are available for Brånemark and IMZ implants.

When correctly positioned, the clip does not grip the cylinder. A small clear-

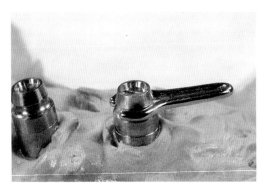

Fig 4-2 a *Sheffield clip fitted to earlier Nobel-pharma gold cylinder.*

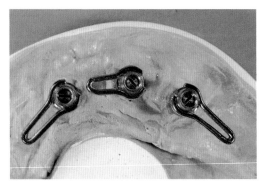

Fig 4-2 b *The tags are located in the most convenient position relative to each other and to the cylinders.*

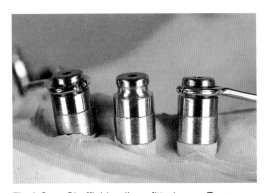

Fig 4-2 c *Sheffield clips fitted on Temporary Retention Cylinders.*

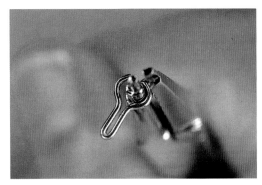

Fig 4-2 d *The retainers are made using orthodontic spring forming pliers.*

ance provides a passive clip location in its groove at rest. This changes to an active contact on a displacing denture movement. A positive resistance results and an audible click is heard when the prosthesis is inserted in the mouth.

After bending with orthodontic spring forming pliers (Fig 4-2 d), the clips are secured in place on the cylinders with plaster. Material which when removed from the processed denture also provides a necessary outward clip movement clearance. Denture base resin contacts

the top of the gold cylinders so a denture settling clearance is not provided.

When the distance between implants is restricted, clips can be rotated to bring their tags into the most convenient position relative to other tags and other cylinders. The same re—positioning can also be used to bring tags into thicker and more convenient denture parts.

When correctly provided, Sheffield clips are compact and protected by surrounding resin (Fig 4-2 e). A displaced Bråne-mark gold cylinder attached to an abut-

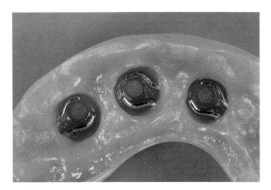

Fig 4-2 e *Sheffield clips incorporated in an overdenture.*

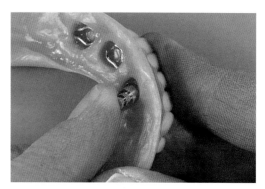

Fig 4-2 f *Displaced replica/gold cylinder showing the range of movement when the clip is still in contact.*

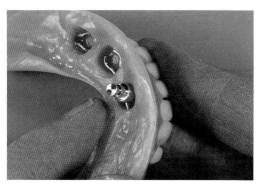

Fig 4-2 g *Clip has realigned the displaced cylinder.*

ment replica shows the range of movement possible with the clip still engaging its retention groove (Fig 4-2 f). Upon release, the clip acts to re—align the cylinder which in the mouth re—positions a displaced denture (Fig 4-2 g).

TEMPORARY COMPONENTS (c)

Temporary and intermediate prostheses may be made using Nobelpharma temporary components as their foundation.

Made from polymeric materials, these comprise an entirely separate four component prosthetic sub—system for the Brånemark implant. Through the use of these components temporary and intermediate prostheses, ranging from single crowns up to and including complete dentures may be made as follows:

● **Prosthesis with contained temporary cylinders.** Prosthesis installed by direct connection to titanium abutments with standard gold screws.
● **Prosthesis with contained temporary tubes.** Prosthesis installed by cementation onto temporary cylinders already gold screw connected to titanium abutments.
● **Prosthesis with contained cast framework with incorporated temporary tubes.** Prosthesis installed by cementation onto temporary cylinders already connected to titanium abutments by gold screws.
● **Resin crown with contained temporary cap.** Restoration installed by cementation over a CeraOne abutment.

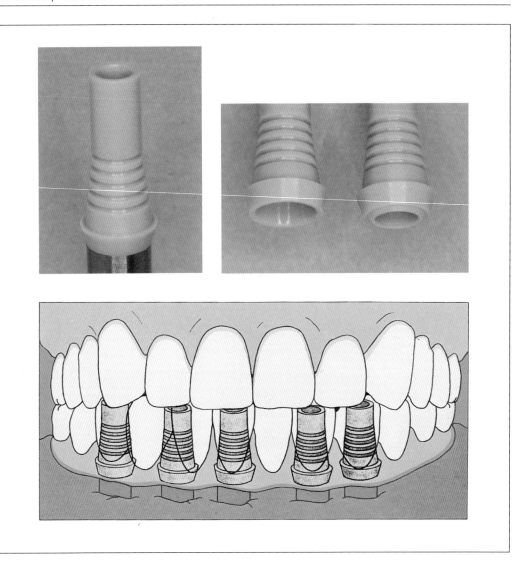

Fig 4-3 a (above left)   *Plastic temporary cylinder gold screw connected to a titanium abutment.*

Fig 4-3 b (above right)   *Fitting surfaces of temporary cylinders. Left for connection with angled and EsthetiCone abutments, right for standard abutments. Note horizontal resin finishing ledge.*

Fig 4-3 c (bottom)   *Screw retained acrylic resin complete prosthesis incorporating temporary cylinders.*

Resin single tooth restorations for the CeraOne abutment are made using a prefabricated cap with an internal hexagon as its foundation. Temporary cylinders form the basis of restorations comprising two or more teeth up to and including complete prostheses. Temporary cylinders are available in two types, one for standard abutments the other for EsthetiCone and angled abutments and are connected in the mouth using standard gold screws (Figs 4-3 a and b).

Temporary cylinders

Made from thermo–plastic poly ether etherkeotne, the cylinder has an extension which forms a gold screw access tube. The height of this can be reduced as necessary with either a stone, disc or bur. Although cylinders do not form a chemical bond with denture base resins, they are mechanically retained by encircling undercut grooves and a horizontal shoulder provided at the skirt makes a neat denture base to the cylinder finishing edge. Without metal reinforcement all resin implant supported prostheses lack strength, so high strength denture base materials may be required for larger more highly stressed prostheses (Fig 4-3 c). Unlike prostheses containing metal frameworks, where the gold cylinders are fixed in their correct positions, dentures containing individual plastic cylinders must be processed on their master cast if cylinder positions are to be accurately recorded in the denture.

The greatest inter–fixture misalignments tolerable by cylinders is 30°. Greater between–implant tilting than this and the cylinders will not fit the abutments.

CONSTRUCTION OF A BRIDGE FOR THE ESTHETICONE ABUTMENT

Depending on clinical use, these may be in the form of either temporary or intermediate restorations.

The best appearance will be obtained when there is a close fitting between the necks of crowns and the soft tissues. A contact which is also necessary if the pre–formed mucosal shape achieved by the healing cap is to be maintained. This technical responsibility is made easier when the model contains a resilient 'mucosa–replica' of these tissues. Soft Gi–Mask material (d), placed in the impression before model casting, makes an effective and durable soft surround to the abutment replicas.

Having first been connected to the abutment replicas with gold screws, the plastic cylinders are reduced in height as necessary to easily clear the opposing teeth. A wax–up of the future teeth and possible trial in the mouth precedes their recording in a Lab Putty matrix (d). Crown and bridge resins applied to the cylinders are then extended incrementally to form the desired bridge. There is no restriction as to the type of autopolymerising, light or heat cured materials which may be used.[5] Before the restoration is finally stained and polished, metal polishing protection caps (c) are screw connected to the fitting surface of each cylinder. The connecting surfaces of cylinders are easily damaged by contact with grinding and polishing wheels, the damage which may occur makes the use of these caps essential.

During the final inspection, abutment cylinder and under prosthesis access may be tested with brushes of the type used by patients for cleaning.

Temporary cylinder skirts are 1.50 mm wide and, depending on soft tissue thickness, restorations can sometimes show these at tooth necks. Fortunately, cylinders have an accommodating neutral colour which is not usually obtrusive (Figs 4-4 a–i).

Temporary tubes

The versatility of temporary cylinders is increased by the use of temporary tubes. Made from clear acrylic resin, the tubes fit

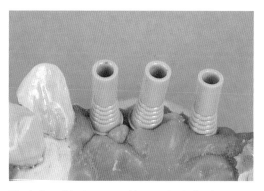

Fig 4-4 a *Master cast with attached plastic temporary cylinders.*

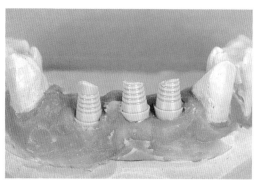

Fig 4-4 b *Cylinders reduced in height to accommodate opposing teeth.*

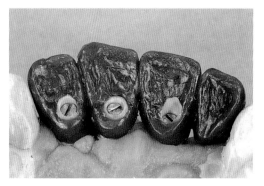

Fig 4-4 c *Trial wax—up of restoration with incorporated cylinders.*

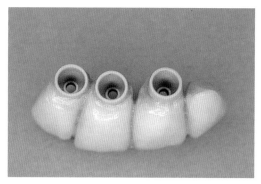

Fig 4-4 d *Bridge showing the abutment connecting surfaces of temporary cylinders.*

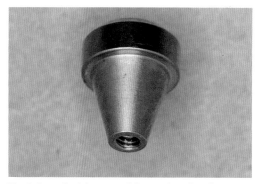

Fig 4-4 e *Stainless steel Protection Cap for covering the fitting surfaces of conical cylinders during finishing procedures.*

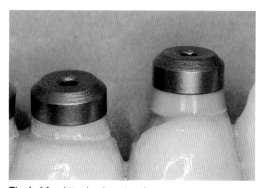

Fig 4-4 f *Attached protection caps.*

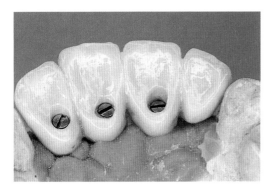

Fig 4-4 g *Finished acrylic resin bridge.*

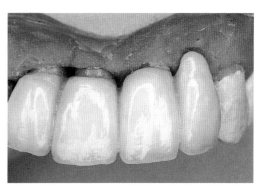

Fig 4-4 h *Appearance of tooth necks showing some cylinder skirt.*

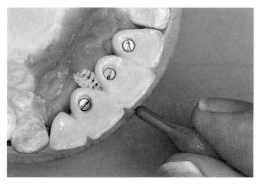

Fig 4-4 i *Testing under–bridge cleaning access with the small brushes which will be used by the patient.*

over temporary cylinders which have been reduced by grinding to the height of their uppermost groove. This makes a removable coping in the manner of a telescope crown (Figs 4-5 a and b). Temporary tubes form a strong bond with denture base and tooth resins to form the basis of an all resin prosthesis which is cemented in place over temporary cylinders installed in the mouth. The grooved cylinder sides provide an additionally

secure cementation, while tubes themselves are easily re–shaped by grinding to provide clearance with adjacent and opposing teeth.

Tubes burn away during mould heating so can be included in patterns as part of cast temporary frameworks. These provide prostheses with gold screw fixation and strength sufficient for longer periods of use. Fitting accuracy is as crucial in temporary frameworks as it is in final prostheses if implant and bone stress overload are to be avoided. Since they do not contain gold cylinders, temporary frameworks may be melted and the alloy used again withouth difficulty or loss.

Through the added versatility of tubes, all resin prostheses can be cemented in place or framework reinforced and screw retained in the mouth as clinically indicated or mechanically necessary.

Cemented bridges can be correctly seated in the mouth only when the angles formed between tilted implants are less than 15°. A screw retained prosthesis with contained cast framework will allow 30° of implant misalignment before connection difficulties are encountered.

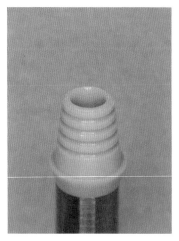 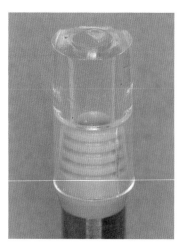

Fig 4-5 a   *Cylinder reduced in height to the uppermost groove. Compare with Fig 4-3 a.*

Fig 4-5 b   *Temporary tube fitting over reduced cylinder.*

CONSTRUCTION OF A CEMENTED TEMPORARY BRIDGE

Temporary cylinders are reduced in height to their top groove before being attached to replicas with standard gold screws. The access holes are then closed with wax (Fig 4-6 a). Tubes placed over the cylinders are then checked for fit and contact with opposing and neighbouring teeth, with interferences ground away as they are found.

When the bridge is designed to replace anterior teeth a wax–up of the proposed restoration precedes the making of a Lab Putty two–part mould. Autopolymerising, heat cured or light cured resin materials are applied directly onto the tubes and form a strong bond. The applied material may partially flow into the screw access holes, which is desirable. These holes are not required in cemented bridges and

their closure provides added strength, particularly of the occlusal surfaces. Crown form shells or temporary crowns may also be used, and simpler restorations made as necessary (Fig 4-6 b). The polymerised bridge may then be stained and polished with the fitting surfaces of the cylinders protected by metal polishing caps.

Installation

The cut–down cylinders are gold screw connected to the abutments in the mouth and the screw access holes again filled with wax. The bridge is then cemented in place over the cylinders (Fig 4-6 c).

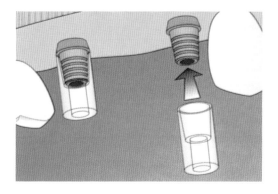

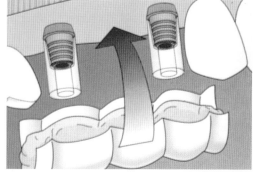

Fig 4-6 a (above)   *The cut—down temporary cylinders are gold screw connected to the abutment replicas and wax placed in the screw holes. A temporary tube is then placed over each cylinder.*

Fig 4-6 b (above right)   *A bridge made of acrylic resin securely bonds onto the tubes.*

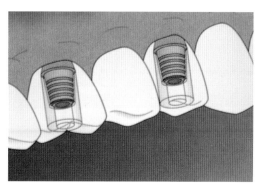

Fig 4-6 c   *All acrylic resin temporary bridge cemented to place in the mouth.*

CONSTRUCTION OF SCREW RETAINED PROSTHESES WITH CAST FRAMEWORKS

Intended for long—term bone conditioning usage as intermediate prostheses, and for temporary prostheses in situations of high functional stress, screw retained prostheses contain an all—cast framework. Because temporary tubes burn away in investment moulds, they can be incorporated into patterns to form a framework connection with shortened temporary cylinders. The frameworks are made entirely from one casting alloy, and gold cylinders are not used. Consequently, re—melting and re—casting is easily achieved without metal loss.

The cut—down cylinders are attached to abutment replicas using guide pins of sufficient length to protrude through the attached tubes. A framework is then made in type 4 gold alloy by the methods described in Chapter 7. This may be made as a simple beam or built—up to full tooth contour and cut—back to accept a veneering of tooth resin. As necessary, the temporary tubes are altered by grinding, to remove unnecessary bulk or tooth contacts (Figs 4-7 a and b).

After casting and finishing, the framework is checked for fit on cylinders still attached to the master cast. If this is satisfactory the cylinders are removed from the cast, coated with luting cement and immediately replaced into the framework. After this, and before the cement has set, the assembly is returned to the model and

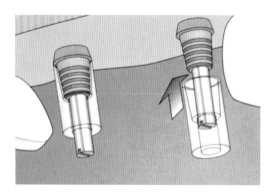

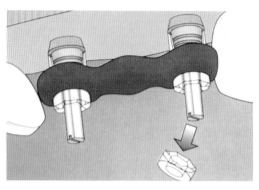

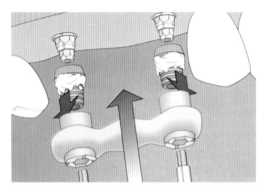

Fig 4-7 a (above left) *The temporary cylinders are reduced as shown in Fig 4-5 a and attached to the replicas with guide pins. The pins then protrude through the seated tubes.*

Fig 4-7 b (above right) *Dura Lay sub-frame before the addition of wax. The tubes are ground as necessary to avoid unwanted tooth contacts.*

Fig 4-7 c *The cylinders are cemented into the framework before guide pin connection of the whole assembly to the replicas.*

the guide pins tightened in place (Fig 4-7 c). When all is set and secure, the resin teeth and other parts are added, followed by staining colouration and polishing.

CONSTRUCTION OF A SINGLE TOOTH USING THE TEMPORARY CAP

The temporary cap is essentially a smaller version of the Nobelpharma metal–ceramic plastic pattern, but with added external retention elements. This trans-lucent polyester cap amounts to a thimble which fits over, and is cemented to, the CeraOne abutment.

Primarily intended for use at the chair-side, its retention tags are reduced in size sufficiently to be incorporated into a pre-fabricated resin crown form or temporary crown filled with self–curing resin. In the laboratory, crown and bridge resins are applied directly onto the cap and shaped to form the temporary tooth. Nobelpharma claim that a chemical bond occurs be-tween the cap and acrylic resin, which is not the case. A sufficient amount of reten-tion elements must be retained in order to provide an adequate mechanical reten-tion for autopolymerising resin materials (Figs 4-8 a–d).

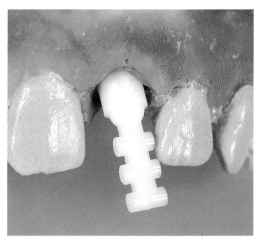

Fig 4-8 a *Polyester temporary cap pushed onto a CeraOne abutment replica.*

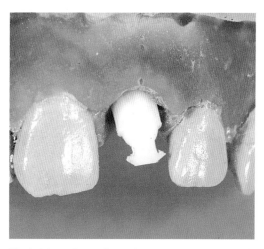

Fig 4-8 b *Retention elements reduced to fit within the future crown.*

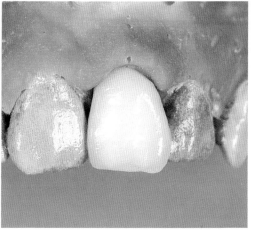

Fig 4-8 c *Finished temporary crown with necessary close fitting adaptation of the tooth neck to the mucosa.*

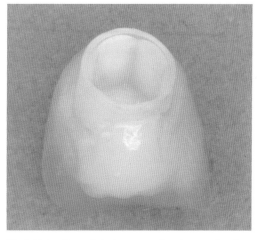

Fig 4-8 d *Completed crown showing protruding cap with internal fitting hexagon.*

REFERENCES

1. Brånemark P-I, Zarb G A, Albrektsson T. Tissue-Integrated Prostheses: Osseointegration in Clinical Dentistry. Quintessence Publishing Co, Inc Chicago, USA, 1985.

2. Henry PJ, Bishop B M, Purt R M. Fiber-reinforced plastics for interim restorations. Quintessence of Dental Technology, 1990/1991. Volume 14. Quintessence Publishing Co Inc. Lombard, Illinois, USA.

3. CeraOne Abutment – Esthetical Single Tooth Replacement. Publication PRI 183 91.02. Nobelpharma AB, Gothenburg, Sweden.

4. Personal Communication. Barry Cayless-Smith, Regent Dental Limited, Leighton Buzzard, UK.

5. Manual Temporary Solutions for Brånemark System Rehabilitation. Publication PRI 264 92.02. Nobelpharma AB, Gothenburg, Sweden.

CHAPTER 4: MATERIALS AND EQUIPMENT

Manufacturer	*UK Agents*
(a) SR-Ivocron-PE	
Ivoclar AG	Ivoclar-Vivadent Ltd
FL-9494 Schaan	44 Boston Road
Liechtenstein	Beaumont Leys
	Business Centre
	Leicester
	LE4 1 AA
(b) Temporary Retention Cylinders	
Implant Innovations Inc	Innovative Dental
1897 Palm Beach Lakes Blvd.	Products Limited
West Palm Beach	Lower Icknield Way
FL 33409	Longwick
USA	HP17 9RZ
(c) Temporary Components	
Protection Cap, conical type DCA 143	
Nobelpharma AB	Nobelpharma UK Ltd
Box 5190	Nobel House
S-402 26 Gothenburg	Packet Boat Lane
Sweden	Uxbridge
	UB8 2GH
(d) Gi–Mask	
Lab–Putty	
Coltène AG	Coltène (UK) Ltd
Feldwiesenstraße 20	8a Teknol House
CH-9450 Altstätten	Victoria Road
Switzerland	Burgess Hill
	RH15 9LF

Chapter Five

The Design of Frameworks for Complete Prostheses

Implant supported prostheses essentially comprise three parts: a cast metal framework to provide strength and rigid connection to its implant/bone bed foundation, artificial teeth, and denture base resin to join the teeth to the framework.

Unlike the cementation of bridges where some natural tooth movement accommodation of slight misfitting may be expected, osseointegrated implants do not move. Consequently, the fitting accuracy criteria required by implant supported prostheses are more exacting than those usually required for bridges.

THE SHEFFIELD FITTING TEST

Frameworks are attached to Brånemark implants by means of small gold screws. In addition to a complete absence of rocking before screw connection, a searching test for the passive fitting of frameworks requires the use of only one gold fixing screw. It must be possible for a single screw to be fully tightened in place in a cantilever abutment replica or cantilever abutment cylinder without any visible discrepancy between any other framework to implant connecting part. In the laboratory this will be tested under times 20 magnification. Loupe magnifiers will assist with the same test at the chairside.

FRAMEWORK DESIGN

When frameworks are contained within the boundaries of a group of implants, an easy opportunity exists to evenly distribute functional occlusal loads over the implants and supporting bone. This is not the case in most edentulous jaws. Because of an anterior placement of fixtures, which avoids the mental nerve, mandibular frameworks usually require distal extension cantilevers to carry sufficient posterior teeth. There are arbitrary recommended cantilever lengths of up to 20 mm in the mandible and usually less in the maxilla.[1-5] The effect of different cantilever lengths on the longevity of implants, supporting bone and frameworks is not known.

The objective of prosthetic treatment is not the usual one of replacing as much of the lost tissues as possible. It is rather to provide a durable prosthesis which satisfies appearance, speech and functional needs and which preserves its implant and bone bed foundations. The response of a prosthesis to functional loads depends on its shape and mechanical properties, together with the behaviour of its bone foundation in resisting the applied load via the fixtures. Masticatory forces cannot be altered, but the manner of their collection and transmission to the jaws is a function of the prosthesis and especially the framework design.

SAFE BEARING

Framework design is usually based on the premise that bone is rigid and that this requires a rigid framework. Although some bone deformation in function must occur,[6] the assumption is equivalent to ignoring any differential fixture/bone movement under load. Occlusal forces collected by the prosthesis must be dispersed over a sufficient number of implants and area of supporting bone to provide a safe bearing. The situation is decided by the number and position of installed implants and bone quality. When the condition of these foundations are less than ideal, safe bearing is more difficult to arrange. Within these factors, safe bearing is obtained through a rigid framework, with the necessary control of cantilever length and size of occlusal table.

Structural engineers cautiously warn that cantilever lengths exceeding one third the inter–fixture distance may reduce the margin of safe bearing. Unfortunately, with recommended fixture separation distances of approximately 8 mm measured between their centres, the resulting cantilever length would be of little practical value. Longer cantilevers are usually required, with a special consideration of their design necessary if bone overload, cantilever and implant internal screw fractures are to be avoided.

FRAMEWORK MATERIALS

Although various framework dimensions have been recommended,[1-5] none of

these have been given in relation to the mechanical properties of individual casting alloys or alloy types. The contrary also applies. Stellite and silver–palladium alloys, metal–ceramic and type 3 and 4 gold alloys have each been proposed, but without framework dimensions.[1-5] Also relevant is the fact that dental alloy manufacturers are unaware of the strength and other mechanical properties required by implant supported frameworks.[7]

PRINCIPALS OF FRAMEWORK DESIGN

Fixture length and bone quality

Cantilever length should reflect the number and length of installed fixtures, together with the quality and maturity of their bone bed. Long fixtures in dense mature bone will provide the best foundation, short ones in poor quality novice bone the least favourable support. It may be necessary in more difficult circumstances to construct intermediate or novice prostheses which will be worn during the immediate post osseointegration or novice bone maturation period (Chapters 4 and 8). Novice bone of lesser quality may be compromised by exposure to full loading, so posterior teeth with reduced occlusal tables are necessary, with increased final dimensions some time later.

Whatever their healing period, some fixtures will always be less–able load bearers. For example, a short fixture installed over the mental nerve will be less able to tolerate loads than longer fixtures installed elsewhere in the same jaw. Similarly, maxillary bone and all grafted bone will require a longer bone maturation period before exposure to full functional loading, while fixtures installed in tuberosities will be in permanently poor quality bone.

Masticatory loads

Because prostheses act to collect occlusal loads and transmit this to the implants and bone, the likely magnitude of this stress forms an important consideration in framework design. A masticatory load of between 33 N and 53 N may be expected from the opposition of natural teeth, fixed bridge or implant supported prosthesis, with a likely maximum biting force of between 94 N and 236 N.[8] When these loads fall onto denture parts situated immediately over implants one situation will apply. When loads fall onto distal extension cantilevers the strain reactions resolved in the framework and implants will change. These strains may be calculated and a typical situation of five mandibular implants installed anterior to the mental nerve is considered (Fig 5-1).

ANALYSIS OF MASTICATORY LOADS

Skalak/McGuire theorem

Skalak[9] assumed frameworks were rigid and that movement in the system occurred only in the bone and implant foundations. Using Skalak's formula derived from McGuire,[10] the vertical loads/reactions at each implant position were determined, assuming load P at the end of one cantilever.

When the ends of 13 mm long cantilevers are loaded, cantilever implants are seen to receive a compressive load of over twice the applied load. Except for implant number 5, which is also under

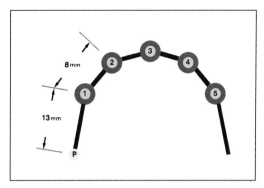

Fig 5-1 Schematic representation of five correctly separated implants connected by a framework carrying 13 mm distal extension cantilevers.

compression, the remaining implants are under varying tensile loads. By these calculations implant number 3 is under a tensile load of approximately twice the applied cantilever load (Table 5-1).

Finite element analysis

As confirmation of these results, a finite element study of the interaction between a prosthesis and Brånemark implants was undertaken.[11] By this method, objects to be studied are geometrically modelled

Table 5-1 *Forces resolved in 5 implants and host bone from a perpendicularly loaded 13 mm cantilever.*

	Implant Position (see Fig 5-1)				
	1	2	3	4	5
Skalak	+2.38	−0.13	−1.91	−0.68	+1.34
Patterson et al.	+2.68	−1.74	−0.62	−0.12	+0.75

Table 5-1 Forces acting on implants from cantilever loading. The + values represent compression, − values tension. Loads expressed as a proportion of load applied.

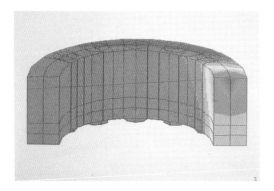

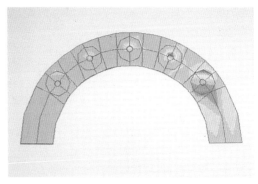

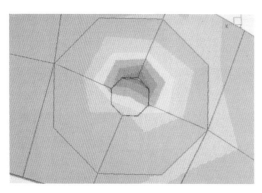

Fig 5-2 a (above left) *Finite element computer representation of an implant supported prosthesis.*

Fig 5-2 b (above right) *Distribution of applied cantilever load. Blue shading represents compression, red shading tension.*

Fig 5-2 c *Computer enlargement of gold screw head in implant Number 2 showing load detail.*

as a connecting network or mesh of elements. All elements are connected at their nodes and it is these connections which are essential to the progressive numerical calculations that take place throughout the model. These calculations produce data on the displacement of each node and hence data of stress, strain, and reaction forces can be deduced by a computer. The computer model was constructed using the implant/framework geometry previously used for Skalak's mathematical method (Fig 5-1), and bore a stylised resemblance to a prosthesis consisting of a heat strengthened type 4 gold alloy framework supporting acrylic resin teeth and denture base (Fig 5-2 a).

When a cantilever loading was simulated, the computer responded by reveal-

ing the position of the resolved loads (Fig 5-2 b). What was shown was that implant number 2 and its internal screws was under the greatest tensile load (Fig 5-2 c), a finding which is at variance with that obtained using the Skalak/McGuire theorem (Table 5-1).

Castigliano's theorem

Again using the framework dimensions and implant configuration shown in Fig 5-1 and Castigliano's mathematical theorem, Patterson and Johns[12] assumed a framework comprised entirely of straight parts. What was indicated was that implant number 2 was under the highest tensile load by an amount approximate to Skalak's prediction for implant number 3

Table 5-2 *Loads resolved in implants and host bone under a 50 N perpendicular cantilever load.*

	Implant Position (see Fig 5-1)				
	1	2	3	4	5
Skalak	+119	−6.5	−95.5	−34	+67
Patterson et al.	+134	−87	−31	−6	+28.5

Table 5-2 Loads resolved in implants and host bone under a 50 N perpendicular cantilever load. The + values represent compression, − values tension. Values expressed as a proportion of load applied.

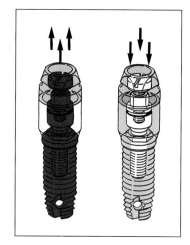

Fig 5-3 *Implants under compression (blue) transmit load to bone without loading the internal screws. Implants under tension (red) load the internal connecting screws and bone.*

(Table 5-1). The flexibility of the mandible under load was not taken into account by any of the studies, so all are comparable in this respect. Patterson *et al.* speculated that the calculated implant loads would be higher if bone distortion was included.

When these load ratios are used with known biting forces (Table 5-2), opposing teeth exerting 50 N would be resolved as a compressive load of 119 N (Skalak) and 134 N (Patterson *et al.*) acting on the cantilever implant. The same biting force would be resolved as a 95.5 N tensile load applied to implant number 3 (Skalak), and one of 87 N to implant number 2 (Patterson *et al.*).

A maximum biting force of 236 N described by Haraldson *et al.*[8] applied to a 13 mm cantilever would theoretically be resolved as a compressive force of 561 N on the cantilever implant and a tensile load of 450 N on implant number 3 (Skalak). This would change to a compressive load of 632 N on the cantilever implant and one of 410 N on implant number 2 (Patterson and Johns).

It is known that gold and titanium implant connecting screws can loosen and fracture in use.[1,3,4,13,14] Since the screws in implants under compression are not

stressed, it may be supposed that it is those screws under tension which are mostly at risk. Compressive loads are conveyed to bone via implants whose individual parts are brought together into even tighter congruity without stressing the screws.

Tensile loads, by contrast, can only load bone in as far as the ultimate tensile strength of the gold and titanium screws holding the implant parts together allow (Fig 5-3).

Conclusions

Emerging from this work, is the explanation of how occlusal loads collected by cantilevers are transmitted to other framework parts to stress implants and their bone bed (Figs 5-4 a and b). Although variables such as actual biting force, the amount and quality of bone, fixture

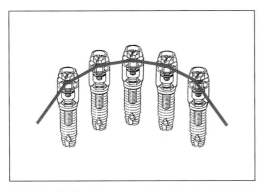 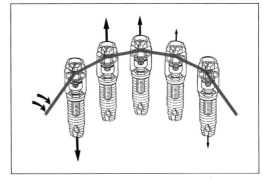

Fig 5-4 a (left)   *A framework (red line) with distal extension cantilevers connected to five implants.*

Fig 5-4 b (right)   *A loaded cantilever applies different loads to implants depending on their position relative to the cantilever.*

lengths and their positions decide the clinical consequences of framework transmitted loads, some guidance for obtaining safe bearing may be obtained. Other factors being equal, the shorter the cantilever the less the transmitted load.

GOLD SCREW PRE–LOAD

Knowing that gold screws can fracture in use, dentists may choose not to fully tighten the screws with the intention of providing a margin of protection. This has a detrimental effect and exposes screws to potentially destructive functional loads. Screws should be tightened sufficiently to stretch them just short of their yield point. A torque of 15 Ncm, preferably from a pre–set torque wrench, provides a manufacturer recommended tensile pre–load of 300 N on the screw which will elastically deform 12 µm under this stress.[15]

The Nobelpharma Torque Driver (DIA 250) and the more recent Nobelpharma electronic Torque Controller (DEA 020) are pre–set to 10 Ncm, this, however, may indicate an unpublished change in required torque.

The mechanism by which correctly tensioned screws are protected from further tensile loads up to the value of the applied pre–load may not be immediately obvious (Fig 5-5). Through complete tightening, screws are protected and their service life extended.[12] A final, correct pre–load is not obtained at the first tightening. Screw settling and partial loss of pre–load occurs after exposure to functional loads, so screws must be re–tightened after a period of use. The settling occurs in three places, under the screw head, between the gold cylinder and the abutment, and in the screw threads. Due to micro–movement between these parts, which reduces microscopically small high spots, settling will be greater with flexible weak frameworks.[15] A higher relative movement between parts can mean that settling is more prolonged, requiring several screw pre–load tightenings. Stiffer frameworks reduce this effect and framework rigidity is an important design consideration.

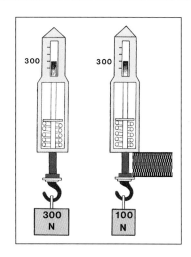

Fig 5-5 *When a theoretical spring balance is loaded by 300 N, a gold screw (shown in red) is also tensioned by 300 N. If a block representation of a framework is interposed between the screw head and balance, then the balance still shows a tensile load of 300 N on the screw shank even if the weight is removed. Any attached weight of less than 300 N will not loosen the clamped block or alter the indicated load of 300 N. The gold screw and spring balance does not recognise any weight or weight fluctuation of less than 300 N.*

CASTING ALLOYS AND INVESTMENTS

Framework manufacture for most implants consists of casting—on to prefabricated gold alloy [platinum alloy] cylinders. Consequently, casting alloys must be chosen on the basis of their thermal properties relative to the cylinders, as well as their mechanical properties. Similarly, casting investments cannot be properly chosen until a casting alloy's melting range is known.

Nobelpharma standard gold cylinders and the conical cylinder for the angulated abutment both have melting ranges of 1280 °C to 1350 °C. An obvious prerequisite, therefore, is that the temperature of cast molten alloy does not closely approach the solidus temperature of the cylinders. An important related consideration is that alloys must be heated to a casting temperature which is above their liquidus temperature. Alloys must be superheated sufficiently, to allow the melt to enter and completely fill the mould before cooling solidification occurs. Superheat-

ing must not be confused with overheating which is deleterious. In practice the difference is a narrow one.

The actual superheating temperatures used by technicians when casting has relevancy if gold cylinder thermal damage is to be avoided.

Control of alloy temperature

Dental technology is unusual in retaining the art of estimating the temperature of molten metal by its emitted colour. Having first shown the ease by which yellow casting gold alloy could be overheated using natural gas and compressed air flames, White[16] investigated the accuracy by which colour—temperature is estimated under normal dental laboratory production casting conditions.

It is known that the brightness of an object in relation to the surrounding visual field plays an important part in visual perception. Bright objects seem brighter when placed against a dark background. Realising that casting machines may be sited in a dimly lit part of the laboratory or near a window in sunlight, White measured the ambient illuminance falling onto six casting machines situated in six different laboratories. Measurements were taken at each casting machine during the morning, noon and late afternoon periods over one day, at one calendar month intervals for one year.

The overall range of measured illuminance ranged from 4000 lux to 100 lux. Illuminance with one machine varied between the extremes of 4000 lux and 265 lux over the year and by as much as 3000 lux in one day. The most consistent machine had an illuminance which did not vary by more than 140 lux throughout the year. The mean of the highest levels of illuminance measured at each machine equalled 1500 lux. The mean of the lowest levels of illuminance equalled 200 lux.

Melting type 4 gold alloys

Using the obtained mean levels of illuminance, White invited a group of 10 qualified technicians to individually flame melt and visually assess the casting temperature of an alloy with a melting range of 860 °C to 940 °C using emitted colour temperature control. The melting crucible had been provided with a miniature thermocouple connected to a remotely positioned temperature indicator which could not be seen by the participating technicians. Three temperature assessments were made under both illuminance levels with 5 minutes between each assessment.

Results

Experienced technicians

The mean and median superheat temperatures achieved by this group under 1500 lux illumination were 19.2 °C and

17.5 °C respectively with six underheating miscast melts. The number of miscasts (25 %) suggests an increased difficulty of estimating temperatures under bright light. The mean and median superheat temperatures under 200 lux illumination were approximately 9 °C higher at 27.9 °C and 27 °C respectively with two underheating miscasts (8.4 %).

The technicians were individually able to demonstrate a very accurate temperature control but these were strongly 'personalised' temperatures. Subject 1 had the widest temperature range with a spread of 25 °C over three melts under 1500 lux. The remaining subjects controlled at least one series of three melts with a tolerance better than 8 °C. This represents a consistency better than 0.85 % of the superheated alloy temperature.

Inexperienced technicians

Although the sample group comprised qualified technicians, subjects 9 and 10 were not usually employed on gold casting.

They were observed to be much less proficient at temperature control, which included an increased sensitivity to ambient lighting. Their performance varied between the extremes of the equivalent of three under–heating miscasts with one participant, to substantial overheating by the other (Table 5-3).

The overall temperatures achieved by the entire group of technicians indicate that the likely casting temperatures to be expected in practice would be within the range of 744 °C to 1162 °C, which is a temperature difference of over 400 °C. The range of casting temperatures used by experienced technicians differed by approximately 70 °C.

Table 5-3 *Estimated casting temperature of a flame melted alloy with a liquidus temperature of 940°C under 1500 lux and 200 lux ambient illuminance.*

Experienced subjects	Illuminance used (lux)	Temperature achieved during three melts (°C)		
		1	2	3
1	1500	935*	955	960
	200	995	977	995
2	1500	950	950	950
	200	945	940*	950
3	1500	938*	944	941*
	200	946	947	949
4	1500	945	940*	948
	200	954	953	955
5	1500	970	1000	1007
	200	980	1000	1000
6	1500	967	967	966
	200	974	972	973
7	1500	969	971	972
	200	972	988	988
8	1500	951	964	962
	200	959	962	956
Inexperienced subjects				
9	1500	1135	1162	1044
	200	1020	1010	1039
10	1500	863*	946	941*
	200	991	927*	980

* Denotes the equivalent of an under–heating miscast.

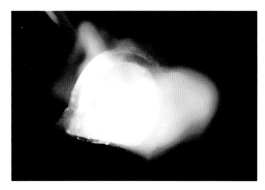

Fig 5-6 *Appearance of molten dental alloy at approximately 1410°C.*

Metal–ceramic alloys

These materials are recommended for frameworks despite the fact that in many instances they have liquidus temperatures close to, if not exceeding, the solidus temperatures of Nobelpharma standard and conical gold cylinders. The practical difficulties of estimating the casting temperature of high temperature alloys has also been described.[16]

The amount of radiant energy emitted by the majority of metal–ceramic alloys heated to casting temperature is sufficient to cause painful eye discomfort to the viewer, together with a retinal after–image which may persist for several minutes. It is impossible to see the surface of the molten alloy with the naked eye (Fig 5-6). Little exists in dental literature regarding suitable eye protection for viewing molten high–temperature alloys. Although some workers and alloy manufacturers have recommended welding goggles, without specifying the colour or visual density required.

When seven experienced technicians were invited to select a British Standard welding filter which would eliminate dazzle and still allow the surface of a pool of molten metal held at 1410°C to be easily seen, all observers preferred British Standard filter shade Number 5 GWF. This filter has a visual density of Dv 1.71.

Wearing goggles with the preferred filters the same seven technicians attempted to identify the correct casting temperature of an alloy with a liquidus temperature of 1310°C. This temperature is 40°C below the liquidus temperature of Nobelpharma standard and conical gold cylinders and 150°C below the solidus

Table 5-4 *Estimated casting temperature of a metal-ceramic alloy with a liquidus temperature 1310 °C using BS Number 5 GWF welding filters.*

| Subject | Temperature achieved during three melts (°C) | | |
	1	2	3
1	1560	1570	1610
2	1340	1365	1350
3	1435	1400	1420
4	1295*	1337	1365
5	1325	1350	1340
6	1365	1360	1352
7	1370	1335	1340

* *Denotes the equivalent of an under–heating miscast.*

temperature of the EsthetiCone gold cylinder. Each technician melted alloy using an oxygen/propane flame adjusted to personal preference and three separate temperature assessments were made (Table 5-4).

Results

Of the 21 temperature estimations, and ignoring the single under–heating error of subject 4, only six melts were below the liquidus temperature of Nobelpharma standard gold cylinders. All three melts of subject 1 exceeded the liquidus temperature of EsthetiCone cylinders. Subject number 1 (melt 3), was seen to use a casting temperature which was 285 °C greater than subject 5 (melt 1).

Conclusions

This data gives some indication of the actual superheating temperatures which may be expected in practice and of the wide variation in temperature control between technicians. The higher superheat-

ing temperatures and greater between–technician casting temperature variation applying when flame–melting metal–ceramic alloys is also shown.

Because of this variation and the need to adequately superheat casting alloys without closely approaching the melting range of the gold alloy cylinders, casting alloys for use with Brånemark standard and angled abutment gold cylinders should not have a liquidus temperature much above 1000 °C. Even with this precaution, skill in temperature estimation is still needed if gold cylinder damage is to be avoided (Figs 5-7 a–c).

The choice of alloy for frameworks

Frameworks must be contained within prostheses of a smaller size than conventional complete dentures, so frameworks themselves need to be as conveniently small as possible; a requirement which will also reduce cost if the alloy is a precious one. Frameworks also need to be strong and fatigue resistant. They can break or deform in use and this has been reported as a treatment complication.[1,4,17] Many otherwise promising high strength casting alloys have the disadvantage of high liquidus temperatures and low percentage elongation. These considerations taken complete indicate the use of a heat treatment strengthened type 4 yellow gold alloy.

Although its resistance to fatigue failure was not available, Stabilor G casting alloy was selected (a). This yellow gold alloy, which has a melting range of 860 °C to 940 °C, has been in continuous and exclusive use at the University of Sheffield School of Clinical Dentistry since 1985 and has been used for national and international courses which have been given there.

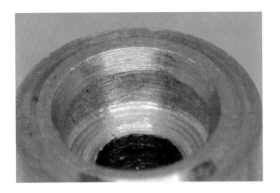

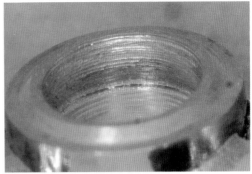

Fig 5-7 a (above)   *Appearance of an unused gold cylinder showing machined fitting surfaces.*

Fig 5-7 b (above right)   *Appearance of a gold cylinder correctly incorporated into a framework by casting—on.*

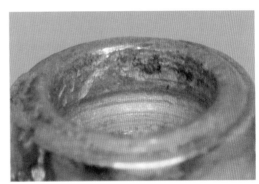

Fig 5-7 c   *Gold cylinder damaged by contact with molten metal.*

CASTING INVESTMENTS

It is probable that alloys with a liquidus temperature of approximately 1000 °C will have solidus temperatures of 80 °C to 90 °C lower. Since the cooling contraction of cast metal is closely related to its solidus temperature to room/mouth temperature cooling range, the thermal contraction of alloys melting at approximately 1000 °C can be adequately compensated by the expansion of gypsum—bonded investment materials.

The higher the solidus temperature the greater the contraction of the alloy on cooling and the greater the compensatory investment expansion which will be necessary (Fig 5-8 a). When cast molten metal has filled the mould, its first contrac-tion is caused by a loss of superheat. This is simply compensated by a reduction in height level of the still fluid alloy. As cool-ing continues between the liquidus and solidus states, a sufficiently thick sprue or added reservoir provides a supply of molten metal to the contracting semi—soft casting. This mechanism avoids contrac-tion porosity in the casting but provides it in the sprues.

The final contraction of the now solid casting from its solidus temperature to room/mouth temperature can only be compensated by the expansion of the investment mould (Fig 5-8 b). Investment materials which have been found to give accurate expansion for the cooling con-traction of Stabilor G gold casting alloy are given in Chapter 7.

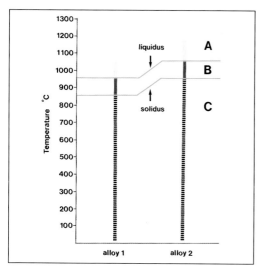

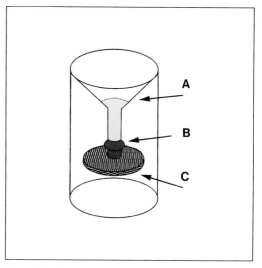

Fig 5-8 a *The contraction of alloys is related to their cooling range. Alloy 1 will require less compensatory investment expansion than alloy 2 because its solidus temperature is lower. The yellow line A) represents superheating, the red line B) the melting range and the black line C) the solidus temperature to room temperature cooling range of the solidified casting.*

Fig 5-8 b *Schematic representation of a cooling cast mould. A loss of superheat results in a lowering of the head of still molten metal A). The liquidus to solidus cooling contraction is compensated by a thick sprue/reservoir B) supplying molten metal to the solidifying casting. The solidus temperature to room temperature contraction can only be compensated by an expansion of the investment mould C).*

STRENGTHENING HEAT TREATMENT

Most alloy manufactures recommend the double return of type 4 gold alloy castings to the furnace, first to homogenise anneal, then to strengthen. An advantage of Stabilor G alloy is that this typical form of heat treatment is not required. Because only sprue removal is necessary in correctly made frameworks and a relatively small area of the casting requires polishing, annealing is not necessary.

Mandatory heat treatment strengthening is simply obtained by allowing the cast mould to completely cool in air to room temperature before removing the casting. Nothing else is necessary. The mechanical properties which then apply

are those given in Chapter 14, under slow cooling (Manufacturers data).

THE FATIGUE RESISTANCE AND STRENGTH OF SHEFFIELD FRAMEWORKS

The resistance of dental casting alloys to stress fatigue is not provided by manufacturers. This important property must be known before the long–term reliability of distal extension cantilevers can be assured. When making decisions about framework dimensions for strength and longevity these must reflect the mechanical properties of the material used for their construction. Also provided must be a wide margin of safety with regard to the

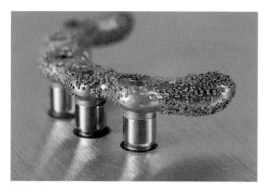

Fig 5-9 a *A Sheffield framework connected to five implants contained in an aluminium plate.*

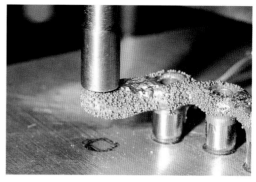

Fig 5-9 b *A ram applying a load of 10 N to 100 N and return five times each second.*

ability of cantilevers and other framework parts to withstand transient heavy biting forces.

Using an epoxy resin adhesive, five 12 mm long replica Brånemark implants were fixed in position 4 mm apart in a 12 mm thick aluminium plate. Fixture ends were aligned flush with the base of the plate so that compressive loads arriving on the implants would be carried by a supporting steel test–bed and not the adhesive (Fig 5-9 a).

Fatigue resistance

A cast Stabilor G framework satisfying the Sheffield fit test and carrying two 13 mm distal extension cantilevers was made using the dimensions, materials and methods described in Chapter 7. The framework was tightened to place using slotted flat headed gold screws pre— loaded from a Nobelpharma mechanical torque wrench. The final arrangement of the implants and framework essentially duplicated that shown in Fig 5-1.

A ram in contact with one cantilever continuously applied a cyclic loading of 10 to 100 Newtons and return five times each second (Fig 5-9 b). The maximum load selected represented approximately twice that of usual mastication with natural teeth.[8]

Strain gauges attached to each abut-ment and underside of the stressed canti-lever were placed with the intention of detecting possible permanent deforma-tion of these parts (Fig 5-9 c). At 10 176 000 load cycles the experiment was termi-nated, since there was no detectable deterioration in any part of the system.

If the obtained fatigue resistance is clin-ically relevant, it represents a situation whereby a Sheffield framework can with-stand a cantilever loading from opposing natural teeth, equal to maximal biting force in some patients[8] once a minute, 15 hours a day for over 30 years, with-out deterioration. The gold screws were shown to be equally fatigue resistant.

Strength

After this test the apparently undamaged gold screws were removed and a new set installed under the same tightening condi-

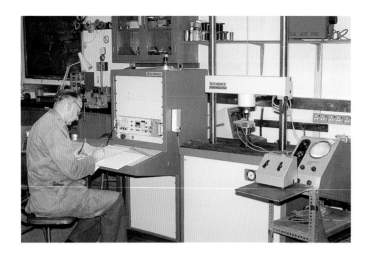

Fig 5-9 c *Test apparatus consisting of fatigue machine, data recorder and oscilloscope monitoring the dynamic condition of the stressed framework.*

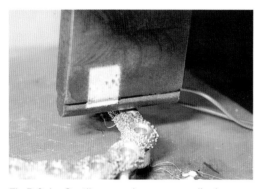

Fig 5-9 d *Cantilever under a perpendicular compressive load.*

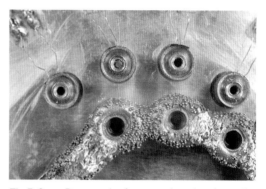

Fig 5-9 e *Removed framework showing the broken gold screw remnant in implant Number 2.*

tions as before. The same cantilever was then subjected to an increasing compressive load until failure occurred (Fig 5-9 d). At a load stress of 1270 Newtons, which is approximately 25 times usual biting force,[8] the gold screw in implant number 2 fractured and the test was terminated (Fig 5-9 e). The position of this failure confirmed the Brook-Smith[11] finite element study and the mathematical predictions of Patterson and Johns.[12] Gold screws have been described as intentionally weak,

fail—safe devices, protecting implants and bone from excessive loading.[14,19] This view is not supported by this test.

From the results of these findings it may be assumed that gold screws will not loosen or fracture when in clinical use. Unfortunately, they sometimes do. Published literature and the availability of proprietary broken screw recovery devices also attest to this fact.

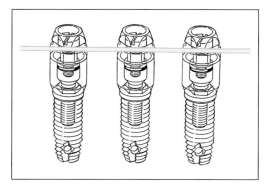

Fig 5-10 a *Accurately fitting framework screw connected to three implants.*

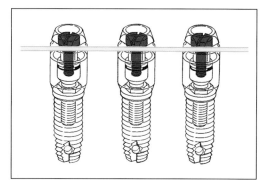

Fig 5-10 b *A tightening pre—load applied to the gold screws places them in tension and clamps the framework to the abutment cylinders. The system is otherwise stress free.*

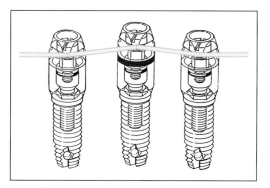

Fig 5-10 c *A framework with a misfitting gap between the central gold cylinder and its abutment.*

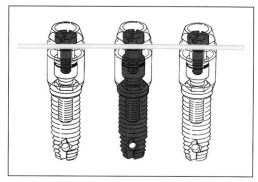

Fig 5-10 d *A tightened central gold screw closes the misfitting gap and applies the tensioning pre—load to the implant and its surrounding bone.*

FRAMEWORK FITTING ACCURACY

The entire literature on implant dentistry insists that a passively fitting prosthesis is mandatory for the long—term preservation of osseointegration. The actual definition of passivity is more obscure. It can be easily demonstrated that a distorted framework or alternatively, a prosthesis containing a distorted framework can be tightened in place to give an appearance of an accurate fitting. Despite this fact careful workers are still deceived by the apparent fitting excellence of screwed—down frameworks.[2,3,5]

When prosthesis to implant fitting gap errors are closed upon tightening in place in the mouth, some of the pre—load applied to gold screws will alternatively be applied to the implants, placing them in tension or compression depending on their position.

In the illustrated example of an accu-

75

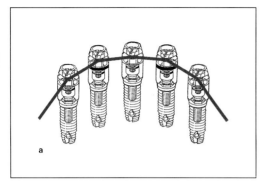

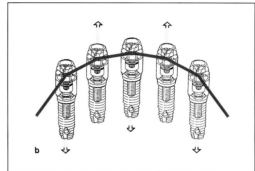

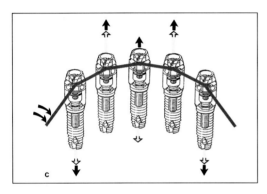

Fig 5-11 *When a framework with the arrangement of framework misfitting shown in a) is tightened to place, the tensile and compressive stresses shown by the yellow lines in b) are continuously applied. When a cantilever is loaded these stresses are increased as shown by the black arrows in c).*

rate and, therefore, passively fitting framework supported by three implants (Fig 5-10 a), gold screw tightening confines the tensioning pre–load to the screws with the effect of clamping the framework and abutment together. The framework, implants and bone are not stressed by this tightening (Fig 5-10 b).

If a gap exists between the central gold cylinder and its abutment, however, (Fig 5-10 c), the pre–load is then applied to the central fixture, placing it and its bone bed in continuous tension (Fig 5-10 d). The forces actually resolved would be more complex than this. The tension produced in the central implant would be accompanied by compressive stresses resolved in the two adjacent implants and their supporting bone.

When cantilevers are bitten on, these intrinsic stresses change. Depending on the number of implants and the location of the misfitting, intrinsic stresses will either be increased (Fig 5-11), or occur in the opposite direction, causing stress reversals in both implants and bone (Fig 5-12). Depending on the severity of these reversals and the quality of the bone, these framework induced stresses may have the propensity to undermine osseointegration.

MISFITTING FRAMEWORKS

Several texts contrast the difference in appearance of an adequately passive fit and an inaccurate fit.[1–3] Misfitting is

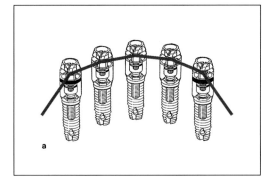
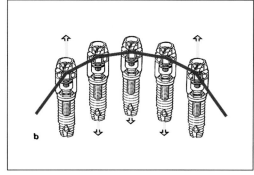

Fig 5-12 *When the framework fitting discrepancies are as shown in a), the installed prosthesis produces the continuous stresses shown by the yellow lines in b). Cantilever loads now have the effect of stressing the implants and bone in the opposite direction as shown by the black arrows in c).*

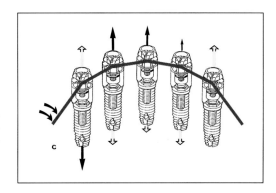

shown as vertical discrepancy gaps between framework gold cylinders and abutment replicas in the laboratory, and the same fault on connection with titanium abutment cylinders in the mouth. On discovering this error the choice is either to remake the defective framework with the risk of repeating the fault, or more usually to divide the casting and rejoin by soldering.

Frameworks made by methods usually requiring soldering corrections,[1-5] or made in pieces to be soldered together[20,21] should be regarded with caution. Apart from increased production costs, the joints are difficult to complete successfully and are usually a source of weakness. The removal of misfitting gaps by framework division and soldering is an expected travail in most described techniques. Also mentioned is the possibility of re—soldering and re re—soldering to eliminate stubborn errors.[20]

Any manufacturer recommended heat treatment strengthening of soldered frameworks carries the possibility of embrittling the joints. Because of these difficulties complete, soldered frameworks are usually fitted in a weak annealed state. An expediency which in turn requires larger, heavier and consequently more expensive castings if adequate strength is to be provided. Larger frameworks are more difficult to cast in one piece, so in turn more soldering corrections are required.

It is the total absence of framework rocking or alternatively the accurate closure of misfitting gaps by soldering which confirms the passive connection of frameworks. No other criteria for identifying a correct fit has been promulgated.

PASSIVELY FITTING ONE—PIECE FRAMEWORKS

Sheffield frameworks are cast in one piece and satisfy the one screw fitting test. Corrective soldering is not required. Since beginning patient treatment with this type of framework in 1985 no fixture or implant part has broken and bone resorption in excess of that described by Strid[22] as minimally usual has not been observed. The materials and technical procedures for framework construction are described in Chapter 7.

ASPECTS OF OSSEO— DISINTEGRATION

Texts devoted to implant failure and bone loss complications have speculated on possible causes. Typically, mechanical overload,[19] undetected framework fitting inaccuracies,[1,4,13,14,23] incorrectly designed bridges[1] and inadequate stress distribution[24] have each been intuitively identified.

Horizontal framework misfitting

Investment moulds are required to expand three dimensionally by an amount sufficient to compensate for the three dimensional contraction of solidified cast metal. At the instant of mould filling the pattern chamber should have been enlarged by an amount which exactly duplicates the imminent contraction of the

alloys solidus to room temperature cooling range.

Providing that the investment mould has been heated in accordance with the manufacturers instructions and the casting made at the recommended casting temperature, mould expansion will be obtained by the inversion expansion of the contained silica. All investments have variable expansion characteristics when they have exceeded their use—by—date, have been stored exposed to the atmosphere and are not mixed with the exactly correct powder/water proportions. Too little mixing water results in over—expansion, too much gives under—expansion, with even small errors having a marked effect.

No investment is equally suitable for all alloys. It is well known that gypsum—bonded materials are not suitable for high—temperature alloys of the metal—ceramic type so must not be used for this purpose. Although phosphate—bonded materials may be used for all casting alloys without mould or casting damage, these materials can provide too much expansion. While it is true that the mixing proportions can be adjusted to achieve different expansions, this is less reliable than materials having predictable performance characteristics without adjustment.

Framework parts, having the largest dimension and the largest bulk, will contract most. In the former this will be the end—to—end framework length and cross—framework size. Dimensions which are unalterable if one—piece castings of the correct size are to be made. Framework bulk is different. Framework enlargement because of weak alloy, those comprising both thick and thin parts, those having ledges, angles and other projec-

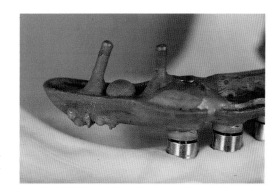

Fig 5-13 *Unfinished heavy silver—palladium alloy framework with supposedly fit—correcting soldered joint. Sheffield one screw test showing continuing misfit.*

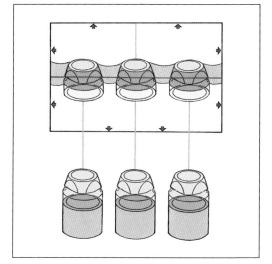

Fig 5-14 a *Moulds must be expanded sufficiently to compensate for alloy contraction if an accurate framework fitting to the abutments is to be made.*

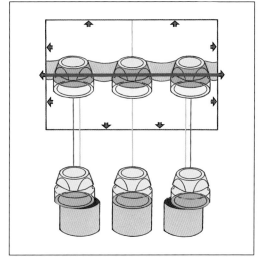

Fig 5-14 b *Moulds can be under or over—expanded. When over—expanded the axial position of the cylinders are not affected but the gold cylinders move apart causing a horizontal misfitting inaccuracy.*

Fig 5-14 c *Gold cylinders are displaced laterally by mould dimensional changes occuring parallel to framework length.*

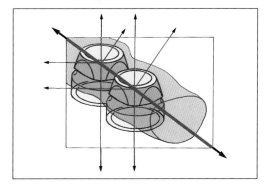

tions from the main framework mass are much more difficult to cast accurately (Fig 5-13).

Sheffield frameworks have a cross—sectional size which allows the gold cylinders to traverse the framework and pierce it with exposed upper and lower rim surfaces. Depending on the position and vertical height of individual clinical abutments, cylinders also occupy the same or nearly the same horizontal level in the pattern, the investment mould and final framework (Figs 7-19 a–f). This regular cross–sectional form and more even distribution of framework bulk reduces the risk of vertical misfitting discrepancies occurring. When moulds are incorrectly expanded it is the distances between gold cylinders which are altered, not their axial position (Figs 5-14 a–c). Through this effect emerges the interesting paradox of a mould expanding in three dimensions, which only affects casting accuracy in two dimensions.

Whatever the pattern chamber's final size at casting temperature, any change of mould dimension will equally affect both the upper and lower borders of the rigid cylinders, so will have no effect on their axial position. Cylinders will be held in place in the same axial position relative to other cylinders, regardless of investment expansion or contraction. An important proviso is that there is not a great disparity of relative axial height in the positions of the cylinders. If cylinders with axial height differences of 1.00 mm are affected by a 2 % framework expansion, then the perpendicular distance increase between cylinders will be only 0.02 mm.

An important additional consequence of over–expansion can be the opening of a space around the cylinder, which is then filled with a flash of metal, so spoiling the fit (Figs 7-20 a and b).

When cylinders are surrounded by more framework metal, necessary in weaker constructions (Fig 5-13), the contracting alloy in thicker framework parts is more able to drag the cylinder with it to cause axial cylinder changes of position and a perpendicular misfit. If the recommended methods of framework manufacture are used, perpendicular framework misfitting will be caused by warped patterns and sprues which connect with each other, not incorrectly expanded moulds. If there is a horizontal casting error of 2 % between gold cylinder separated by 4 mm, cylinder separation will then be 4.08 mm. Since the error is additive, the total error applying over several cylinders would be greater than this.

The effect of horizontal framework misfitting

Using deliberate mould over–expansion, five oversized edentulous frameworks were experimentally made to observe the extent of cylinder separation caused. When these known to be inaccurate castings were returned to the master model from which their patterns were derived, they appeared to fit perfectly. Observed was the contradiction of the passively accurate fitting of known to be inaccurate frameworks. There was no rocking or visible gap between any gold cylinder and abutment replica, but a horizontal displacement between cylinders and replicas was easily apparent (Fig 5-15).

When searching for an explanation for

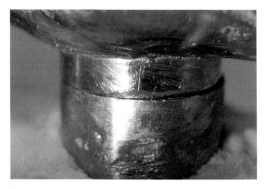

Fig 6-15 *Absence of any vertical fitting discrepancy gap between a gold cylinder contained in a misfitting casting and an abutment replica contained in a master model. Note horizontal fitting error.*

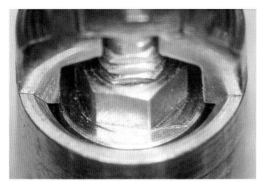

Fig 5-16 a *Accurate connection of a gold cylinder to a titanium abutment cylinder.*

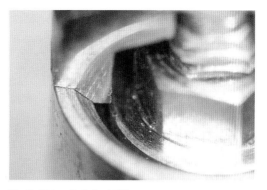

Fig 5-16 b *Detail of fitting.*

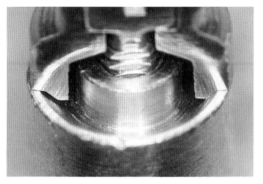

Fig 5-16 c *Lateral misfitting gap of 0.12 mm between a gold cylinder and abutment replica.*

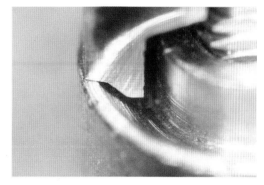

Fig 5-16 d *Detail of misfitting.*

this horizontal fitting error accommodation, 3 mm and 4 mm standard Bråne-mark gold cylinders and a gold screw were sectioned and test fitted to several titanium abutment cylinders, only an accurate connection of these parts was observed (Figs 5-16 a and b). When the same sectioned parts were then connected to Nobelpharma type DCA 015 abutment replicas, a lateral fitting error of up to 0.12 mm between the internal fitting surfaces was seen (Figs 5-16 c and d).

This abutment replica error allowed a horizontal 'float' misalignment to exist be-

tween the connected parts. When sectioned replicas were alternatively fitted to impression copings to duplicate the clinical impression situation, the same horizontal connection error was apparent (Fig 5-16 e). The clinical significance of this finding was revealed by asking several experienced dentists and technicians to screw connect replicas to copings contained in impressions. When the impressions were then sectioned and the connections examined, lateral misfitting errors of up to 0.10 mm were observed (Figs 5-16 f and g).

81

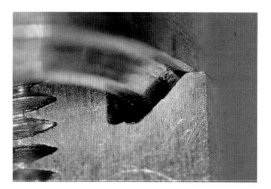

Fig 5-16 e *Sectioned abutment replica connected to an impression coping showing lateral misfitting gap.*

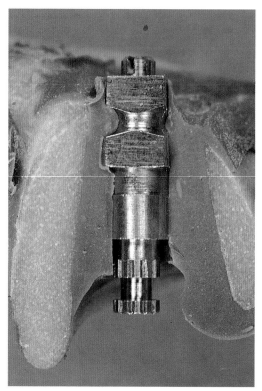

Fig 5-16 f *Sectioned impression showing impression coping to replica fitting. This connection is almost always hidden within impression material.*

Because of this floating fit, abutment replicas placed in an accurate impression could each occupy a laterally displaced position in the resulting master cast. Self—evident is the impossibility of constructing a framework or prosthesis which would accurately fit the patient using such a cast. Crucially important to these findings is that lateral prosthesis to implant fitting errors arising either from inaccurately made frameworks or inaccurate master casts can not be similarly accommodated in the mouth. Framework gold cylinders can only make an accurate connection with titanium abutments (Figs 5-16 a and b).

Fig 5-16 g *Lateral abutment replica to coping fitting error of approximately 0.10 mm.*

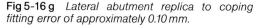

THE CONNECTION ACCURACY OF GOLD SCREWS AND GOLD CYLINDERS

The head and shank diameters of slotted gold screw type DCA 075 were measured and the found dimensions compared with the screw head recesses and screw

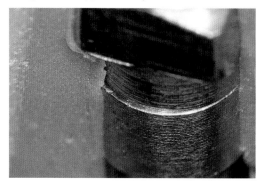

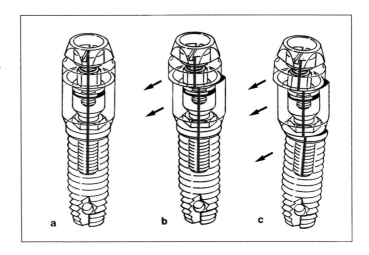

Fig 5-17 a *The correct alignment of the individual parts comprising the Brånemark dental implant.*

Fig 5-17 b *The first effect of a horizontal framework fitting error is to laterally load the gold screw and the bone.*

Fig 5-17 c *In more pronounced lateral fitting errors the gold and abutment screws, the fixture and the bone are loaded to a greater extent.*

shank apertures provided in 4 mm gold cylinders (DCA 072), EsthetiCone gold cylinders (DCA 141), and Angulated Abutment gold cylinders (DCA 103) (Table 5-5).

Results

From Table 5-5 it can be seen that when a gold screw is correctly centred in a gold cylinder, any lateral framework to implant fitting error in excess of approximately 0.10 mm will have the effect of bending the gold screw on tightening. Over or under–expanded cast frameworks, or accurately made frameworks fitting models containing laterally displaced abutment replicas require implants and their internal screw parts to deform on tightening in place in the mouth. This deformation then artfully conceals the error, while the host bone is continuously stressed by the elastically deformed implant (Figs 5-17 a–c).

Depending on the extent and direction of the lateral error, inaccurate frameworks can also stress implants in opposite directions to produce a wedging action (Figs

Table 5-5 *Dimensions of Nobelpharma gold screw (DCA 075) and the internal screw fitting parts of Nobelpharma gold cylinders.*

Gold screw, flat head, slot. (DCA 075)

Head diameter (mm)	Shank diameter (mm)
2.25	1.37

Standard gold cylinder. (DCA 072)

Recess for screw head (mm)	Aperture for shank (mm)	Clearance with screw head (mm)	Clearance with screw shank (mm)
2.58	1.57	0.16	0.10

EsthetiCone gold cylinder. (DCA 141)

Recess for screw head (mm)	Aperture for shank (mm)	Clearance with screw head (mm)	Clearance with screw shank (mm)
2.47	1.54	0.11	0.08

Angulated abutment gold cylinder. (DCA 103)

Recess for screw head (mm)	Aperture for shank (mm)	Clearance with screw head (mm)	Clearance with screw shank (mm)
2.42	1.60	0.08	0.12

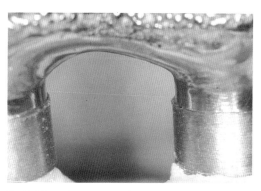

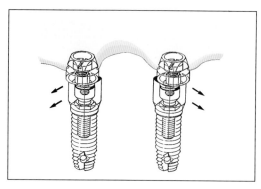

Fig 5-18 a *Over—expanded bridge supported by two implants. Note horizontal ledges indicating the misfitting.*

Fig 5-18 b *Loads resolved in the implants and bone.*

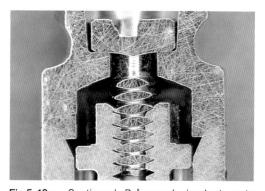

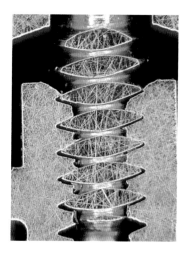

Fig 5-19 a *Sectioned Brånemark implant. note the small lateral clearance between the head of the gold screw and its cylinder.*

Fig 6-19 b *Fitting of the gold screw in the abutment screw. Only four of the seven threads are actually used.*

Fig 5-19 c *The apexes of the abutment screw internal threads form ready fracture sites.*

Fig 5-19 d *Points of fixture weakness occur where the internal threads of the fixture arrive opposite external ones.*

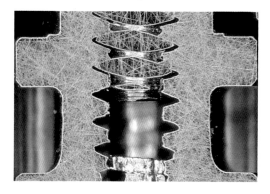

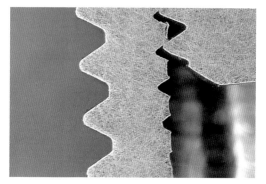

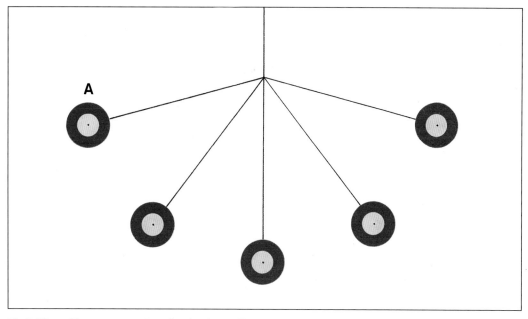

Fig 5-20 a *Discs representing five implants. Place the over and under—expanded frameworks on the transparency over the implants and align gold cylinder 1 with implant A. Note the impossibility of correctly aligning the remaining cylinders.*

5-18 a and b). If these loads occur within the physiological tolerance of the bone then all will be well. If this tolerance is exceeded then the response may be one of accelerated resorption.

Horizontal framework loading begins from the gold cylinder onto the gold screw and abutment. Of the seven threads of the gold screw only four are fully engaged in the abutment screw, so bending readily occurs. Under more severe circumstances the abutment screw is also stressed, with this focused at the apex of one of the internal threads. If the fixture itself is sufficiently deformed, then fixture fracture is likely to occur at some point where the internal threads arrive opposite external ones (Figs 5-19 a–d).

Mechanical engineers assert that when implant parts are correctly aligned, tight-ened and loaded by forces occurring in the mouth, their internal connecting screws should not loosen or fracture.[12, 19] A different situation applies with bent screws. The fatigue strength of deformed screws is significantly diminished with a service life which can be measured in months rather than years.[12]

THE SIGNIFICANCE OF REPLICA ERRORS

Like other lost—wax castings in restorative dentistry it is quite certain that frameworks are made with horizontal as well as the more usually recognised vertical fitting errors. Horizontal errors are not easily removed by those who would divide castings and make soldering corrections. In the instance of a five implant framework, it will be necessary to divide and solder the casting in four places (Figs 5-20 a and b). In frameworks with six connections there must be five corrective joints. The discs shown on page 85 represent implants and their central dots the positions of the threaded holes for the gold screws. If the number 1 cantilever gold cylinder in the over-sized and under-sized frameworks shown on the transparency are superimposed over implant A, the horizontal misalignments applying at other implants are easily observed. Over—expanded or under—expanded frameworks connected at one point act with the effect of compounding the error measured at other framework connection points. This is an important fact.

These cumulative lateral fitting errors deform the implants by an amount easily in excess of that which is minimally necessary to bend the gold screws (Table 5-5). The order by which gold screws may be tightened will have no influence on correcting this fault. By the nature of these errors, the searching nature of the Sheffield single screw fit test is further illustrated and the need for casting accuracy emphasised. The error is caused in three distinctly separate ways:

1. Abutment replicas may occupy laterally displaced positions in impressions on connection to impression copings.
2. Gold cylinders and, therefore, framework patterns may be screw connected to abutment replicas in laterally displaced positions.
3. Gold cylinders may occupy laterally displaced positions in over or under—expanded frameworks.

Horizontal connection errors have been overlooked and virtually every text book

and many illustrated articles in the literature inadvertently show the existence of this inaccuracy in work seen on master casts (Fig 5-21). The error is not seen on work in the mouth unless accompanied by gross additional misfitting (Fig. 5-22). For this to be the case it can be confidently proposed that an implant bending accommodation and horizontal bone loading must have occurred on prosthesis installation.

THE FRACTURE AND LOOSENING OF GOLD SCREWS

When the fracture faces of several obtained gold screws which were fractured in different mouths were examined, all showed crack arrest lines. These lines provide good evidence of fatigue fracture and can record the progress of a crack front as it travels across the shank of the screw (Figs 5-23 a and b). The diminutive final tensile fracture face suggests that the screw was only under a small tensile stress.

It may be speculated that the screw was deformed on tightening and that a crack was initiated at some slight manufacturing blemish in the threads. Functional loads were then sufficient to widen and extend the crack in a direction related to the screws deformation, with the crack front eventually able to almost completely traverse the screw shank before eventual failure. When more highly stressed components have smaller fatigue cracks, they fracture (Figs 23 c and d). Gold screws experimentally fractured by deliberate over—tightening show an entirely different fracture face (Figs 5-23 e and f).

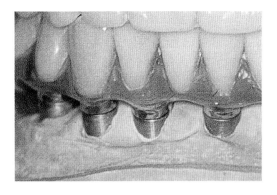
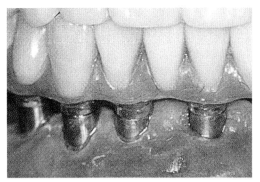

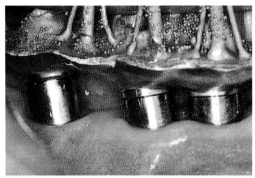
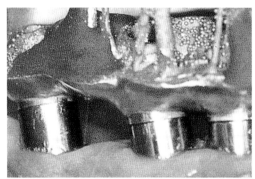

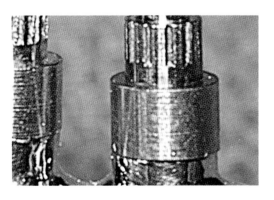
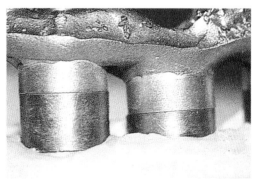

Fig 5-21 *Unattributed illustrations from the literature showing lateral misfitting connection errors between gold cylinders and abutment replicas.*

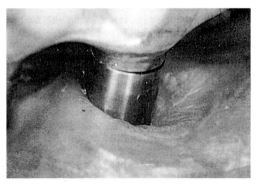

Fig 5-22 *Undetected gross misfitting.*

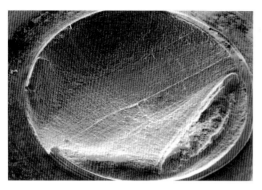

Fig 5-23 a *Gold screw fracture face showing crack arrest lines and small final fracture face.*

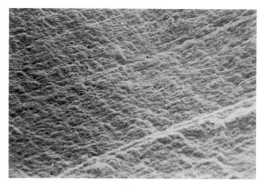

Fig 5-23 b *Detail of crack arrest lines. Width of visible field 180 μm.*

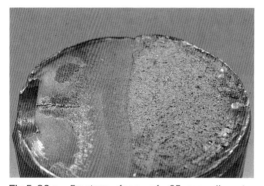

Fig 5-23 c *Fracture face of 65 mm diameter power transmission shaft. A fatigue crack was able to extend half way across the shaft before catastrophic failure.*

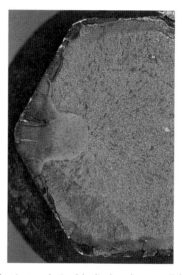

Fig 5-23 d *Fracture face of a 35 mm diameter highly stressed steel bolt showing small fatigue crack sufficient to cause catastrophic failure.*

Fig 5-23 e *Fracture face of gold screw deliberately fractured by over—tightening.*

Fig 5-23 f *Detail of fracture face. Width of visible field 180 μm.*

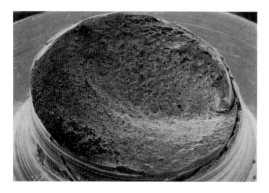

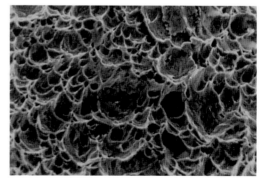

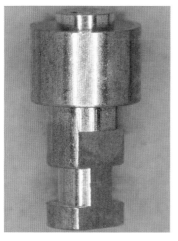

Fig 5-24 a *Improved Nobel-pharma abutment replica for the standard clinical abutment of the Brånemark implant.*

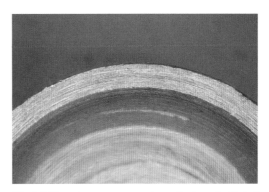

Fig 5-24 b *Appearance of redesigned Nobel-pharma abutment replica fitting surface chamfers.*

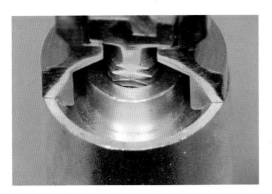

Fig 5-24 c *Connection accuracy of a sectioned gold cylinder with the new replica.*

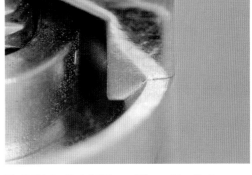

Fig 5-24 d *Detail fitting of the gold cylinder.*

Fig 5-24 e *Sectioned impression coping showing its accurate connection with the new replica.*

Fig 5-24 f *Detail of accurately fitting impression coping and the new replica.*

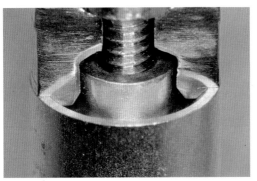

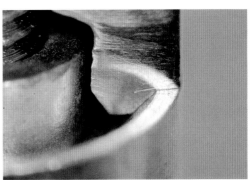

AN IMPROVED ABUTMENT REPLICA FOR THE BRÅNEMARK IMPLANT

Based on the described findings, a new replica was designed by Nobelpharma AB for the Brånemark implant with the objective of improving impression/master cast accuracy and the prevention of horizontal framework fitting error concealment (Figs 5-24 a–f). By use of this replica, the Sheffield single screw fitting test now instantly reveals framework and prosthesis fitting errors.

The new component which replaces the previous one, was first introduced by Nobelpharma AB in late 1990.

ABUTMENT REPLICAS FROM INDEPENDENT MANUFACTURERS

Abutment replicas are internationally available from several independent manufacturers. Twelve Type 186A Brånemark Analogs, [abutment replicas] from a prominent manufacturer were examined for horizontal connection errors with Nobelpharma standard gold cylinders and impression copings. Even with un– aided vision, individual replicas were seen to vary to the extent that no two had the same shape or finish of fitting surface. Some had a rough un–machined appearance, the raised parts of which prevented a complete cylinder to replica fitting (Figs 5-25 a and b).

When Nobelpharma gold cylinders and impression copings were screw connected to these replicas, horizontal fitting discrepancies in excess of 0.20 mm were observed (Figs 5-25 c and d). The replicas had been deliberately made in this way to allow an easy seating of prostheses during technical work in the laboratory.[26] The contrary is necessary.

Alternatively, when 12 type LA200 Standard Lab Analogs from another independent manufacturer (b) were examined, a uniformly accurate and satisfactory connection with Nobelpharma gold cylinders and impression copings was seen (Figs 5-26 a and b).

CONCLUSIONS

After undergoing two surgical operations, numerous visits to the surgery and consulting rooms and waiting for the final prosthesis, patients can become anxious. Clinicians are aware of this and of the importance attached to the installation of the finished prosthesis. These pressures can sometimes act to obscure an objective clinical assessment of technical work. Under these circumstances it can be difficult to deliberately look for technical problems and errors.

Some important aspects of technical work cannot be evaluated at the chairside at all. Whether, for example, the framework has been made from appropriate materials or has been correctly heat treated cannot be seen. Dental technology has important responsibilities here. The future fitting of prostheses by contrast is conveniently assessed at the framework stage using the Sheffield fitting test, while remembering that errors to be found are three dimensional ones. It is better and easier to be critical at this stage than later.

The use of parts and materials important to the preservation of osseointegration and prosthesis longevity on the basis of manufacturer recommendation and not independent evaluation remains unsatisfactory.

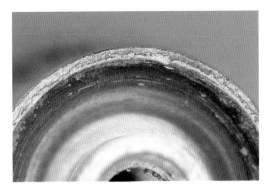

Fig 5-25 a *Unmachined fitting surfaces of an abutment replica from an independent manufacturer. Compare with Fig 5-24 b.*

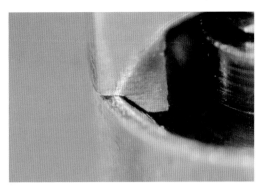

Fig 5-25 b *Nobelpharma gold cylinder raised from fitting contact by abutment replica fitting surface roughness.*

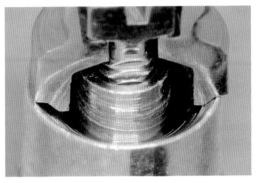

Fig 5-25 c *Horizontal connection error between a Nobelpharma gold cylinder and inaccurate abutment replica.*

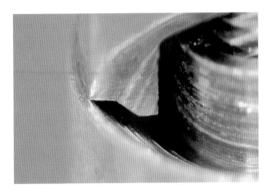

Fig 5-25 d *Detail of lateral misfitting.*

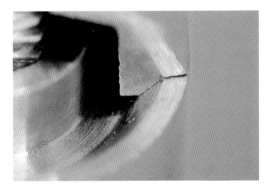

Fig 5-26 a *Accurate fitting connection between a Nobelpharma gold cylinder and an Implant Innovations Standard Lab Analog [abutment replica].*

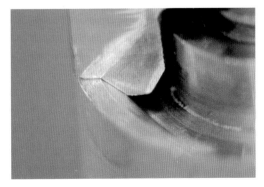

Fig 5-26 b *Accurate fitting of Nobelpharma impression coping with an Implant Innovations Standard Lab Analog [abutment replica].*

FACTORS WHICH MAY AFFECT THE LONG TERM SURVIVAL OF OSSEOINTEGRATED DENTAL IMPLANTS

	Less certain	More certain		Less certain	More certain
1	Natural teeth opposing implants	Mucosa borne denture opposing implants	12	Occlusal table laterally displaced relative to implants	Occlusal table centrally over implants
2	Few implants	More implants	13	Porcelain teeth	Resin teeth
3	Poor quality bone	Better quality bone	14	Passively fitting prostheses	Misfitting prostheses
4	Short fixtures	Long fixtures	15	Short or concealed abutments	Easy cleaning access to abutments
5	Large occlusal table	Small occlusal table	16	Occlusal interferences	Occlusal balance
6	Implants arranged in line	Implants arranged in a curve	17	Horizontal implant loads	Perpendicular implant loads
7	Poor oral hygiene	Good oral hygiene	18	Implants installed with irregular spacing	Implants installed with regular spacing
8	Long cantilevers	Short cantilevers	19	Inaccurately made implant/ prosthetic components	Accurately made implant/ prosthetic components
9	Full loading at earliest confirmed osseointegration	Full loading after confirmed osseo-integration and bone remodelling	20	Laterally stressed implants	Loads transmitted along an implants long axis
10	Novice bone	Mature bone			
11	Bruxist with opposing natural teeth	No para-function with opposing complete denture			

REFERENCES

1. Brånemark P-I, Zarb G A, Albrektsson T. Tissue-Integrated Prostheses: Osseointegration in Clinical Dentistry. Quintessence Publishing Co, Inc, Chicago, USA, 1985.

2. Taylor R L, Bergman G F. Laboratory Techniques for the Brånemark System. Quintessence Publishing Co, Inc, Chicago, USA, 1990.

3. Hobo S, Ichida I, Garcia LT. Osseointegration and Occlusal Rehabilitation. Quintessence Publishing Company, Tokyo, Japan, 1989.

4. Beumer III J, Lewis S G. The Brånemark Implant System: Clinical and Laboratory Procedures. Ishiyaku EuroAmerica, Inc. St. Louis, USA. 1989.

5. Fredrickson E J, Gress M L. Laboratory procedures for an osseointegrated implant prosthesis. QDT Yearbook. 1988. 12: 15–37. Quintessence Publishing Co., Lombard, USA.

6. Hobkirk J A, Schwab J. Mandibular deformation in subjects with osseointegrated implants. *Int J Oral & Maxillofac Implants* 1991; 6: 319–328.

7. Personal communications:
   a) Degussa AG, Frankfurt, Germany.
   b) Engelhard Industries Ltd, Sutton, Surrey, UK.
   c) Johnson Matthey Dental Materials Ltd, Birmingham, UK.

8 Haraldson T, Carlsson G E, Ingervall B. Functional state, bite force and postural muscle activity in patients with osseointegrated oral implant bridges. *Acta Odontol Scand* 1979; 37: 195–206.

9. Skalak R. Biomechanical considerations in osseointegrated prostheses. *J Prosthet Dent* 1983; 49: 843–848.

10. McGuire W. Steel Structures. Prentice—Hall Inc, New Jersey, USA, 1968.

11. Brook-Smith M. The study of fatigue life of small gold locating screw used in osseointegrated implant technique. B Eng thesis, University of Sheffield, 1988.

12. Patterson E A, Johns R B. Theoretical analysis of the fatigue life of fixture screws in osseointegrated dental implants. *Int J Oral & Maxillofac Implants* 1992; 7: 25–34.

13. Gregory M, Murphy W M, Scott J, Watson C J, Reeve P E. A clinical study of the Brånemark dental implant. *Br Dent J* 1990; 168: 18–23.

14. Balshi T J. Preventing and resolving complications with osseointegrated implants. *Den Clin N Am* 1989; 33: 821–868.

15. Jorneus L. Screws and cylinder in the Nobelpharma implant system. *Nobelpharma News* 1987; 1: 7.

16. White G E. The standardisation of variables in dental casting. M Med Sci thesis, University of Sheffield, 1985.

17. Lindquist L W, Carlsson G E, Glantz P-O. Rehabilitation of the edentulous mandible with a tissue integrated fixed prosthesis: a six year longitudinal study. Quint Int 1987; 18: 89–96.

18. White G E. The resistance of selected dental casting investments to casting stresses. PhD thesis, University of Sheffield, 1987.

19. Rangert B, Jemt T, Jorneus L. Forces and moments on Brånemark implants. *Int J Oral & Maxillofac Implants* 1989; 4: 241–247.

20. Faculty of Odontology, The Institute for Applied Biotechnology, Gothenburg, Sweden. Manual for treatment with jawbone anchored bridges according to the osseointegration method. 1985.

21. Lundqvist S, Carlsson G E. Maxillary fixed prostheses on osseointegrated dental implants. *J Prosth Dent* 1983; 50: 262–270.

22. Strid K-G. Chapter 11 Radiographic results, Tissue-Integrated Prostheses: Osseointegration in Clinical Dentistry. Quintessence Publishing Co, Inc, Chicago, USA. 1985.

23. Worthington P, Bolender C L, Taylor T D. The Swedish System of osseointegrated implants: problems and complications encountered during a 4-year trial period. *Int J Oral & Maxillofac Implants* 1987; 2: 77–84.

24. Adell R, Lekholm U, Rockler B, Brånemark P-I. A 15-year study of osseointegrated implants in the treatment of the edentulous jaw. *Int J Oral Surg* 1981; 10: 387–416.

25. Patterson E. Fatigue analysis of gold screws in osseointegrated dental implants. Conference. Problems, Complications and Failures and their Prevention. Malmo, Sweden. 1990.

26. Hill B R, President. Implant Support Systems, Inc., Irvine, California 92720, USA. Personal communication, June 1992.

CHAPTER 5: MATERIALS AND EQUIPMENT

Manufacturer	UK Distributor
(a) Stabilor G casting alloy	
Degussa AG	Degussa Limited
Postfach 110533	Winterton House
D-6000 Frankfurt 11	Winterton Way
Germany	Macclesfield
	SK11 OLP
(b) Standard Lab Analogs	
Implant Innovations	Innovative Dental Product Limited
Suite 117	Wellington House
1897 Palm Beach Lakes Blvd.	Lower Icknield Way
West Palm Beach	Longwick
FI 33409	HP17 9RZ
USA	

Chapter Six
Angulated Abutments

The need for these is self recommending, if not at the time of fixture installation or abutment connection then certainly during laboratory work. Implants can occupy less than convenient positions for prosthetic care. Labial or buccally inclined emergence angles and mutually divergent angles can provide almost insoluble technical problems (Figs 6-1a and b). In extreme cases screw access holes can form ugly notches in the incisal edges of teeth (Fig 6-1c). This frightful appearance, which arises from incorrect fixture position and angulation, cannot usually be mitigated by alternative tooth positioning, no matter how inventive. Having arrived

this far it is inconveniently late to consider re–starting prosthetic treatment with angulated abutments, although this is a last resort option.

Some implant angulations prevent technical work. Prostheses containing standard gold cylinders cannot be connected to implant abutments when their included angles are greater than 30–40° (Fig 6-1d).

These mechanical and aesthetic difficulties can usually be reduced, if not entirely corrected, by the use of angulated abutments to alter the angle of abutment to fixture connection (Fig 6-1e).

The need for angulated abutments and

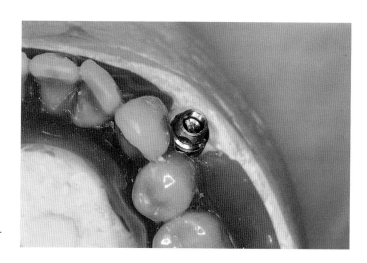

Fig 6-1a   *Standard abutment and gold cylinder located outside the area covered by an overdenture.*

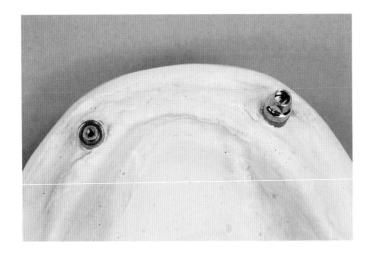

Fig 6-1 b *Relative position of the malplaced overdenture implant.*

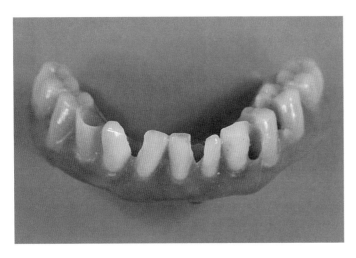

Fig 6-1 c *Gold screw access holes emerging through the incisal edges of teeth forming unsightly notches.*

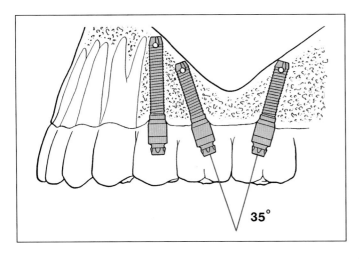

35°

Fig 6-1 d *Implants installed with angles greater than 35–40° prevent the installation of prostheses in the mouth.*

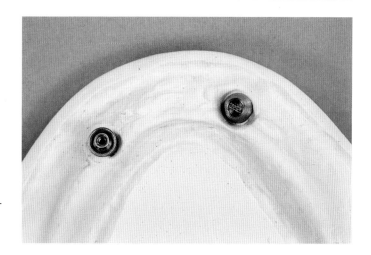

Fig 6-1 e *New improved position of the gold cylinder shown in 6-1b after realignment with an angulated abutment.*

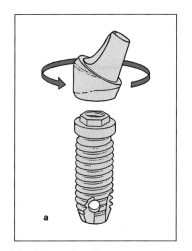

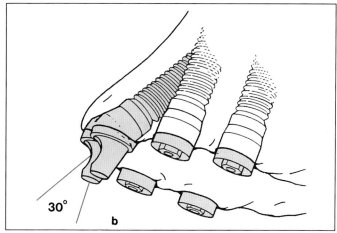

Fig 6-2 a *The abutment can be rotated to connect with the fixture in 12 different positions.*

Fig 6-2 b *The connected abutment forms an angle of 30° to the long axis of the fixture.*

their clinical deployment should occur before commencing prosthetic care. It is disappointing to realise that these are necessary only when technical work is compromised.

THE FUNCTION AND USE OF ANGULATED ABUTMENTS

Standard abutments are linear extensions of fixtures. Alternatively, when angled abutments are connected to standard fixtures they form a rotary 12 position screw joint, each with an angle of 30° to the long axis of the fixture (Figs 6-2 a and b). They may replace standard abutments in either jaw

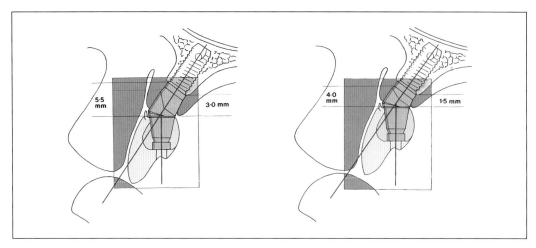

Fig 6-3   *Angulated abutments are used in two collar sizes depending on soft tissue thickness.*

for all prostheses and without restriction, but are not suitable for single implant supported teeth. The lack of an interlock between the gold cylinder and the abutment carries the risk of crown rotation in single implant supported teeth.

Angulated abutments are provided with either 4.0 mm × 1.5 mm and 5.5 mm × 3.0 mm collar heights, the selection of which depends on soft tissue thickness (Fig 6-3). Both types have an abutment cone height of 4 mm with 15° taper which requires a matching impression coping, abutment replica and gold cylinder (Figs 6-4 a–d). The abutment cone and conical cylinder complete has an overall height of 5.5 mm and, despite an appearance to the contrary, the cylinder fits its angulated abutment only at a provided horizontal shoulder. There is no cylinder to abutment contact along its tapered walls (Fig 6-5). Because of this the gold screw has the important additional function of centring the cylinder on its tapered abutment cone.

Conical gold cylinders have the same melting temperature range as standard gold cylinders and are also incorporated into frameworks by casting–on. Unlike standard cylinders, conical ones do not possess an external circumferential groove, which in standard cylinders usefully serves as a framework finishing edge. Consequently, the wax pattern to cylinder margins can be made in different positions, a variation which is used to alter the under prosthesis and abutment cleaning access space as necessary. The finish of the pattern to cylinder junction must be quite perfect. Conical cylinders are thin, so any grinding or heavy polishing of rough framework parts adjacent to the cylinders can drastically weaken them (Figs 6-6 a and b). Because of their lighter construction, conical cylinders are also more easily distorted. The precaution of conical Polishing Caps (a) is mandatory during all framework and prosthesis finishing procedures (Fig 4-4 e).

The conical gold cylinder for the Estheti-Cone abutment is interchangeable with that of the angulated abutment, with the advantage of a higher melting range of

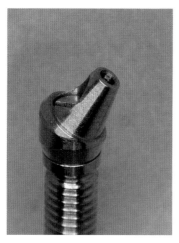

Fig 6-4 a *Fixture with attached angulated abutment.*

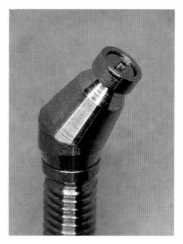

Fig 6-4 b *Angulated abutment with attached gold cylinder.*

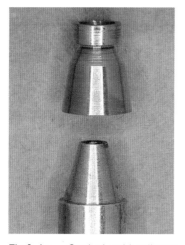

Fig 6-4 c *Conical gold cylinder and tapered abutment replica.*

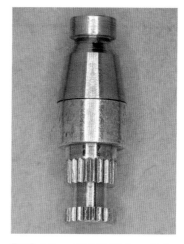

Fig 6-4 d *Connected cylinder and abutment replica.*

1460 °C–1500 °C. This increased temperature range tolerance is useful and necessary when conical cylinders have to be incorporated into metal–ceramic frameworks. EsthetiCone cylinders have the advantage of a schamfer at their marginal rim which gives a finishing edge both to the framework and added ceramic.

Nobelpharma literature sometimes describes the gold cylinder for the angulated abutment as either tapered or conical and the EsthetiCone cylinder as conical. To avoid confusion these cylinders should always be identified by their type numbers (see Chapter 14).

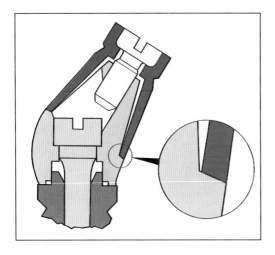

Fig 6-5 *The conical gold cylinder (red) contacts the abutment only at the shoulder.*

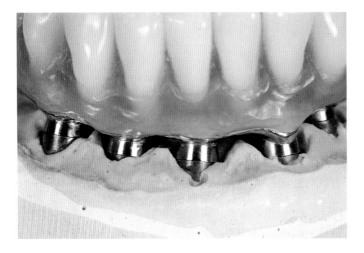

Fig 6-6 a *Prosthesis entirely supported by angulated abutments.*

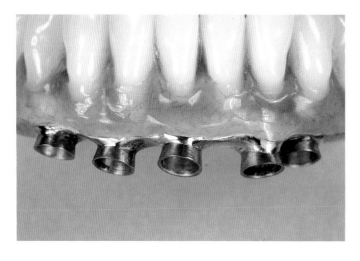

Fig 6-6 b *Conical gold cylinders emerging from framework. Note characteristic trumpet shape.*

CHAPTER 6: MATERIALS AND EQUIPMENT

Manufacturer	UK Supplier

(a) Protection Caps (Type DCA 143)

Nobelpharma AB	Nobelpharma UK Ltd.
Box 5190	Nobel House
S-402 26 Gothenburg	Packet Boat Lane
Sweden	Uxbridge
	UB8 2GH

Chapter Seven
The Construction of a Mandibular Fixed Complete Framework

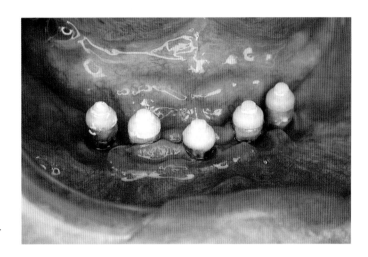

Fig 7-1 a *Clinical abutments with connected protective healing caps.*

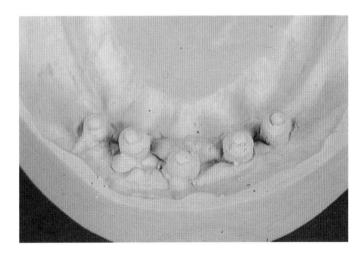

Fig 7-1 b *Primary model showing abutments and healing caps.*

PRIMARY IMPRESSIONS – STUDY CASTS

Primary impressions of both jaws are taken. The obtained study casts are necessary as a diagnostic aid for framework and prosthesis design and for making special trays. The abutment terminals are usually protectively covered at this time and the presence of this cover shown on the cast (Figs 7-1 a and b).

Despite the existence of an otherwise satisfactory upper complete denture, it is almost always better to remake these to the different situation of an opposing implant supported prosthesis.

SPECIAL TRAY CONSTRUCTION

The objective of the final impression is to record the positions of the abutments in the mouth and transfer these to a master cast. When impression copings are incorporated in impressions, they register the individual positions of abutment terminals; an arrangement which allows a master cast to contain abutment replicas which are in the same position as the abutments in the mouth.

The required tray needs to be provided with an aperture for abutment cylinder access. This is made by first placing a wax block former 8 to 10 mm wide and 12 to 15 mm in height over the abutments shown on the study casts (Fig 7-2 a). A sheet of autopolymerising resin dough is then draped overall and trimmed to the required periphery. Special Tray resin has proven to be a satisfactory material for this work (a).

An anteriorly projecting handle serves the additional function of strengthening the tray in an area weakened by its abut-

ment access opening (Fig 7-2 b). There must be a generous tray to coping clearance, together with a tray height which allows future guide pins to protrude through the opening (Fig 7-2 c). Upper trays are made to the same design (Fig 7-2 d).

IMPRESSION MATERIALS

After the dentist has removed the healing caps or other cover, impression copings are connected to the abutments with guide pins. When everything is correctly arranged the pins protrude through the tray opening without tray contact (Figs 7-3 a and b).

Impressions are made in impression plaster as well as in a variety of elastic materials. With thoughts of greater security in mind, some dentists prefer to join copings together in the mouth using Dura Lay autopolymerising resin before taking the impression (b). Others join copings with impression plaster, either in conjunction with other materials, or in a single overall plaster impression. Impressions are removed from the mouth by unscrewing, but not removing, the guide pins (Fig 7-3 c).

Defects such as under or over–extension or small soft tissue blemishes are now of reduced importance, as the future prosthesis will not contact these parts.

PLACEMENT OF ABUTMENT REPLICAS

Abutment replicas are attached to the copings by carefully re–tightening the guide pins (Fig 7-4 a). This ostensibly simple procedure requires careful pur-

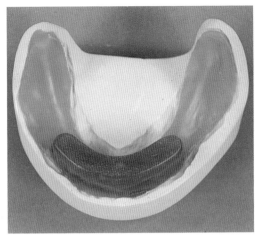

Fig 7-2 a *Wax block former which provides the basis of an abutment access opening.*

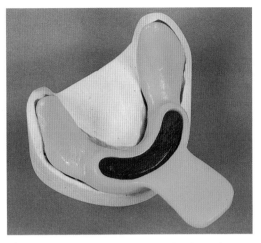

Fig 7-2 b *Finished autopolymerised resin tray with strengthening handle.*

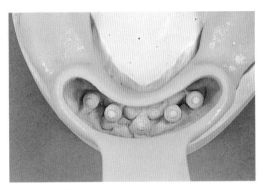

Fig 7-2 c *There must be an adequately wide clearance between the abutments and the sides of the tray.*

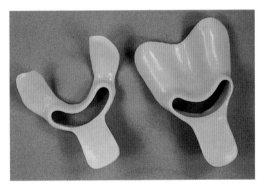

Fig 7-2 d *Mandibular and maxillary trays are made to the same design criteria.*

pose. Any coping movement detected during guide pin tightening indicates a serious error and the impression must not be used. Care must also be taken not to over–tighten pins which can displace erstwhile secure copings.

A concerning factor is the entrapment of unseen impression material between a coping and inserted replica. Plaster scrapings are easily produced during replica insertion and these mischieviously lodge between replicas and copings to cause a connection inaccuracy (Fig 7-4 b). This error is avoided by inserting the replicas twice. Once to reveal and remove plaster debris, the second to correctly tighten the replica in place (Fig 7-4 c).

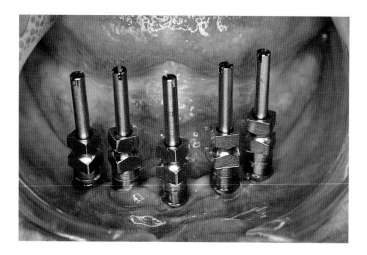

Fig 7-3 a *Impression copings are connected to the abutments using guide pins.*

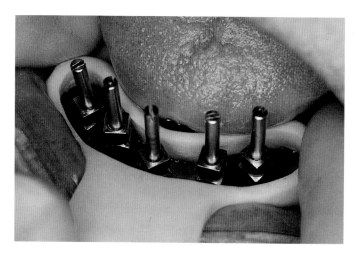

Fig 7-3 b *The screwdriver slots of the guide pins must be accessible with the tray correctly positioned in the mouth.*

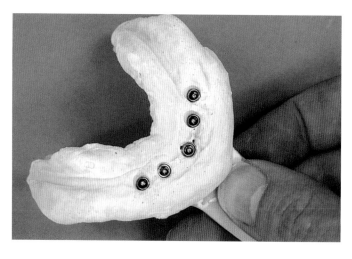

Fig 7-3 c *Plaster impression showing the exposed fitting surfaces of the impression copings which connect with the abutment replicas.*

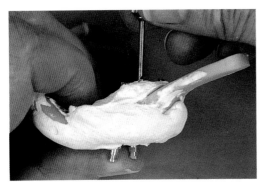

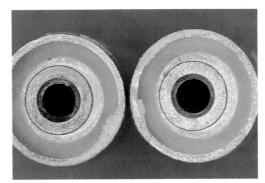

Fig 7-4 a (above left) *Abutment replicas are attached to the copings by carefully re—tightening the guide pins.*

Fig 7-4 b (above right) *Impression plaster scrapings produce replica to coping fitting errors.*

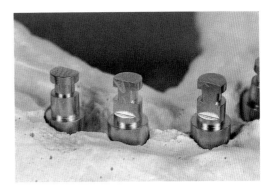

Fig 7-4 c *Plaster impression with abutment replicas tightened to place.*

Fig 7-5 a (left) *Master cast containing abutment replicas in the same positions as the abutments in the mouth.*

Fig 7-5 b (right) *The fitting surfaces of replicas onto which a framework and a prosthesis will be made.*

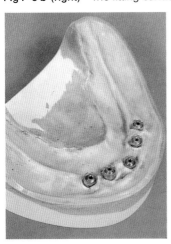

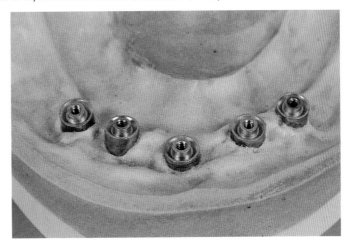

Following replica connection, the cast is poured in hard stone. The guide pins must be unscrewed before the impression can be removed and the cast trimmed (Figs 7-5 a and b). Coping and guide pin parts may now be recovered from the impression and returned for re—use.

THE RE—USE OF COMPONENTS

Except for gold cylinders, which are irretrievably incorporated into frameworks by casting—on, all other parts of prosthetic kit have the potential to be re—used. A possible exception is the abutment replica. This component must exactly replicate the titanium abutment cylinder in the patients mouth if an accurately fitting prosthesis is to be made. Replicas have fitting surfaces which are easily damaged during laboratory work and these should not be used again in impressions. Damaged replicas are always useful for resin processing and some of these should be retained for this purpose. Whether used replicas should be used again in impressions is questionable, and would certainly depend on a $\times 20$ microscope confirmation of completely undamaged fitting surfaces.

The archiving of completed work items including master casts (Chapter 8), has the effect of reducing the availability of used replicas, which on balance is probably a good thing. The best and most consistent work will always be done on new replicas.

FRAMEWORK CONSTRUCTION

In addition to the design considerations discussed in Chapter 5, a crucial prere-

quisite is to make an accurately fitting framework pattern. It is self evident that a casting can not have a better fit than the fitting quality of the pattern from which it is formed. The situation is exactly analogous to a photographic negative and its print. The print quality of a photograph can only be as good as the negative from which it is derived.

Frameworks must also be adequately strong and fatigue resistant in small dimension; qualities which reduce alloy cost and increase space for the artifical teeth. By this design, the need for constructions of an irregular and thereby difficult—to—cast shape is also reduced. In resorbed jaws the prosthetic replacement of lost bone, soft tissues and teeth will require an extremely large denture. In these mouths there will be ample space for frameworks. When the available space is small and/or implants occupy inconvenient positions a diagnostic trial denture may be necessary (See Chapter 8, Method 2).

New teams may care to test—fit their first framework patterns in the mouth. This is a good idea and provides assurances that their impression technique, model and pattern making are accurate before making their first castings. Some texts recommend that successful trial patterns be used to cast the final framework. For reasons described later in this chapter, it is unwise to do this, unless the pattern has been correctively divided between each gold cylinder and rejoined before investing and casting.

PATTERN MAKING

Gold cylinders of either 4 mm or 3 mm height are selected as dictated by avail-

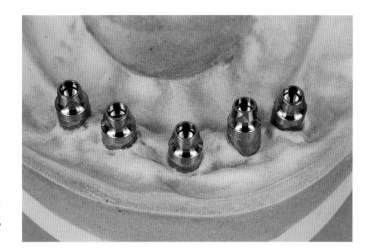

Fig 7-6 a *Gold cylinders are tightly screwdriver attached to the replicas using slave gold screws.*

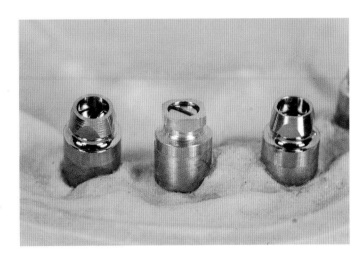

Fig 7-6 b *Three and four millimetre cylinders can be used as necessary to make a more even overall cylinder height.*

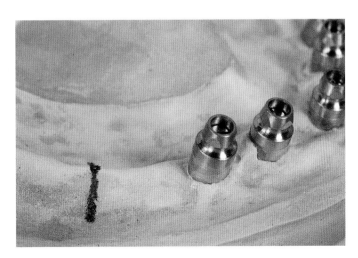

Fig 7-6 c *Pencil mark indicating the extent of a 13 mm cantilever measured from the centre hole of the cantilever replica.*

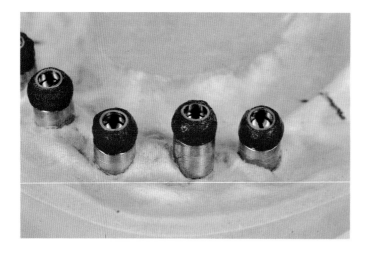

Fig 7-7 a *Resin 'doughnuts' are built—up around each cylinder.*

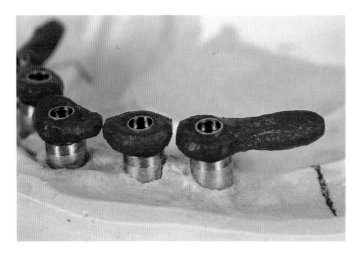

Fig 7-7 b *Cantilevers are added and 'doughnut' parts enlarged until only a small space exists between them.*

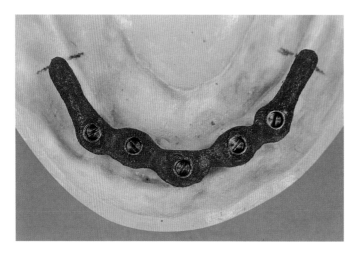

Fig 7-7 c *The parts are required to be joined by only a small amount of connecting resin, a precaution which reduces polymerisation contraction distortion.*

able space and abutment cleaning access considerations. Cylinders of both heights may be used together as necessary to correct individual slight differences in abutment height (Figs 7-6 a and b). Selected cylinders are then securely tightened with a screwdriver to the abutment replicas using short guide pins or slave gold screws as preferred.

If bone quality has been assessed as good and there are five or six installed implants, pencil marks are made on the model at 13 mm distances measured distally from the centre threaded hole of the cantilever abutment replicas (Fig 7-6 c). If the bone is poor and/or 7 mm or 10 mm cantilever fixtures have been installed, then only 10 mm marks and cantilevers are made. When cantilever fixture length varies from one side of the jaw to the other, then cantilever length varies accordingly.

Resin sub—frame

Dura Lay resin is added in increments to form 'doughnuts' around each gold cylinder (Fig 7-7 a). This material extends from the lower border of an encircling external groove to cover the remaining cylinder sides. After polymerisation, further material is added, including cantilevers. This work continues until the individual parts are separated by spaces which are less than 0.50 mm wide (Fig 7-7 b). The intention is to produce gaps which require only a small final mix of resin to join them. By this method resin polymerisation contraction and sub—frame distortion is minimized (Fig 7-7 c).

Alternatively, the sub—frame may be made in one piece before dividing it between the cylinders with a thin disc and joining the parts with Dura Lay as before. If resin flows onto the skirt sides of the cylinder, this material is cut away with a small hot knife.

After final polymerisation do not remove the sub—frame from the master cast or loosen the fixing screws.

Addition of wax

A veneer of hard inlay wax (c) is added to cover the sub—frame. This conceals the resin entirely and forms the final shape of the framework. The final fit of the pattern is more accurate when wax is added almost immediately after polymerisation. The tail of an Ash Number 5 wax carving instrument (d) is conveniently shaped for this work (Fig 7-8 a). The surface contour of the pattern smoothly flows from part to part without sharp angles, projections, flats or concavities. When the framework must make a longer span between cylinders, the pattern rises into an arched form (Figs 7-8 b–d).

Cantilevers emerge from their gold cylinders with a clearance of at least 3.0 mm from mucosal tissue immediately beneath. This or a greater clearance must be maintained along the entire length of the cantilever as measured on the master cast. When this distance cannot be maintained there are two alternatives. If a 1.5 mm to 2.0 mm clearance is possible, the lower half of the cast cantilever can be exposed from resin, have a smoothly rounded form and be polished. If even this reduced clearance is not possible, the distal end of the cantilever may lightly contact mucosa in the manner of a bridge pontic. By whatever method, there must be an adequate cleaning access space distally to the cantilever abutment.

Measured from the upper border of the skirt, the pattern to gold cylinder connec-

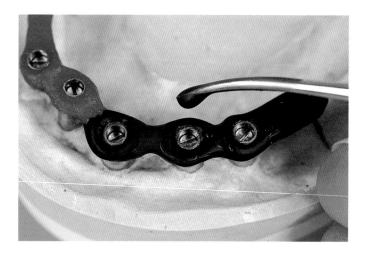

Fig 7-8 a *Hard inlay wax is applied to the sub—frame in small increments.*

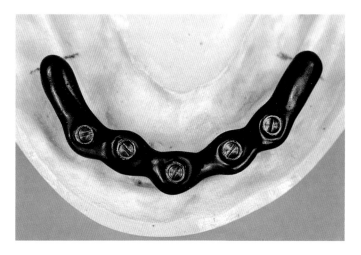

Fig 7-8 b *The finished pattern has a smoothly rounded form with a complete absence of raised ledges, rods, angles and other projections.*

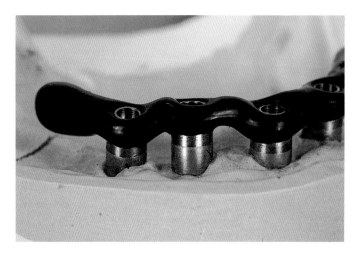

Fig 7-8 c *When the pattern is required to make larger spans between cylinders it rises into an arched form.*

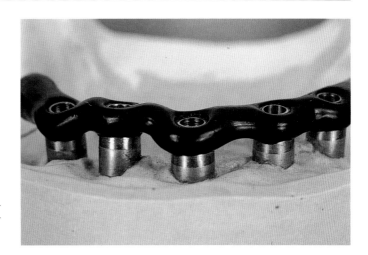

Fig 7-8 d *The pattern may undulate as necessary between cylinders while maintaining its cross—sectional dimensions.*

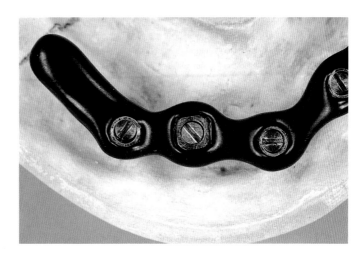

Fig 7-9 *Pattern with 3 mm and 4 mm cylinders showing upper cylinder margins clear of wax and a raised rim of wax encircling the 3 mm cylinder.*

tion will be at the full height of the cylinder in 4 mm cylinders and full height plus a 1 mm wax rim in the case of 3 mm cylinders. This means that the pattern will be 3.00 mm to 3.50 mm high between the cylinders. Wax must not cover any part of what must be an exposed upper rim of gold cylinder if contact of an investment mould wall will securely locate the cylinder within the pattern chamber (Fig 7-9). Between cylinders the pattern is 4.5 mm wide, which is the same diameter as the cylinders. The cross—sectional width of the pattern increases to 6.5 mm as it enlarges to incorporate individual cylinders (Fig 7-10). If because of space limitations a 1 mm rim of extra wax cannot be added above 3 mm gold cylinders, then the pattern must be made 1 mm wider at this point. Cantilevers have a squarer cross—section with 4.5 mm to 5 mm sides and rounded corners.

With the possible exception of the exact site of cantilever connection, wax is not

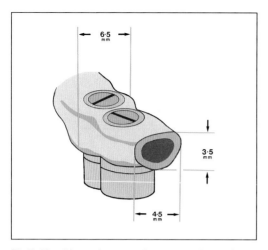

Fig 7-10 *Dimensions and construction of the framework pattern.*

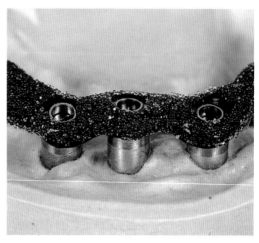

Fig 7-11 *Plastic beads provide an entirely satisfactory resin retention system.*

allowed to encroach onto cylinder skirts. No trace of wax should remain on what must be a scrupulously clean margin of metal. Wax here will encourage a thin flash of cast metal to flow over skirts or worse, onto the cylinders fitting surfaces (Figs 7-20 a and b). The provided dimensions are suitable for Stabilor G type 4 gold alloy. They may not be suitable for other alloys whether strengthened or not.

When all accessible wax work is finished the retaining screws or pins are removed and the framework briefly removed from the cast for a final shaping of its otherwise inaccessible underparts. A final light flaming should quickly achieve an overall smooth, rounded form. Heavy flaming should be avoided, as this may distort the pattern. *Immediately this work is finished, the framework must be returned to its master cast and all screws fully re-tightened.*

Veneer—Lock plastic beads sprayed onto applied liquid adhesive provides an entirely satisfactory resin retention system

(Fig 7-11) (e). Beads are used on the upper half of the pattern and all over cantilevers having a 2 mm or more mucosa clearance. Miniature wax or plastic loops, arrow—heads and other undercut retention aids used in cobalt—chromium work may also be used, provided that they are small and do not materially alter the achieved cross—sectional form and dimensions of the pattern. These aids provide usefully increased retention when the lower part of cantilevers need to be exposed from resin and polished. Rods, framework extension undercut ledges and other projecting parts should not be used. They add unnecessary bulk to the framework and produce a shape which is more difficult to cast accurately.

Because Sheffield frameworks are of small cross—section, resin edges arrive thick and not liable to flaking or lifting. Therefore it is not generally necessary to provide resin finishing gutters, although these can be made providing that they are of the smallest possible size.

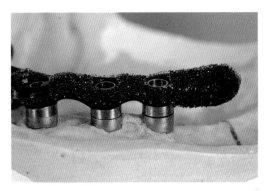 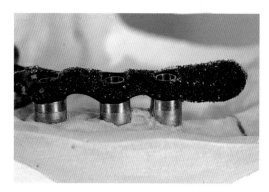

Fig 7-12 a (left) *Pattern showing misfitting gap with remotely positioned single fixing screw.*

Fig 7-12 b (right) *The pattern is left for 16 hours with all fixing screws in place. The same single screw test now shows a perfectly fitting pattern.*

PATTERN STRAIN RELIEF

The completed pattern is not yet ready for investing. The reason for this is easily demonstrated using the Sheffield one screw fitting test. If, immediately after pattern making and bead attachment, all the retaining screws are removed except one in a cantilever replica, the pattern is seen not to fit. It rarely does. Fitting discrepancy gaps will exist between the remaining gold cylinders and abutment replicas (Fig 7-12 a). Alternatively, when a sprued pattern with all retaining screws tightened in place is left overnight or longer, the Sheffield single screw test then shows a perfectly fitting pattern (Fig 7-12 b). Patterns must not be invested until they can demonstrate an accurate fitting. Any production delays which may occur due to the process of testing for pattern strain relief is time well spent.

SPRUING THE PATTERN

The required sprue former length is dictated by casting ring height. A Whip Mix Number 4391 casting ring has a height of 57 mm and a diameter of 64 mm which will conveniently contain most framework patterns. A matching rubber crucible former for centrifugal casting is also available (f). Since patterns must be sited 6–8 mm away from the open end of the ring, each sprue former will be approximately 30 mm long.

Implant supported frameworks are comparatively large and a special consideration of their spruing necessary if contraction porosity is to be avoided. The greatest bulk of metal will be in the cantilevers so these must have one sprue former each. Elsewhere, the pattern is usually of smaller volume, so can have fewer sprues as necessary.

Four 4.0 mm diameter (or wider) round wax sprue formers of equal length are attached full diameter to the pattern. Attachment is on the upper surface of the pattern between the gold cylinders and half—way along the cantilevers. The connection must be made with the wax forming the surface of the pattern. This surface is coated with plastic beads and adhesive, so that sprue formers attached only to this

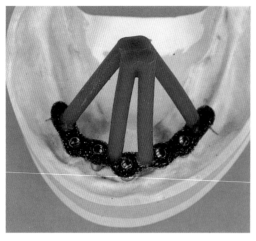

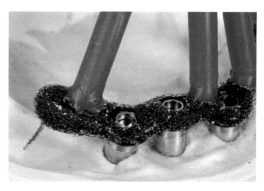

Fig 7-13 b *Sprue attachment is at its full diameter and half way along the cantilevers.*

Fig 7-13 a *Sprue formers of equal length and 4 mm minimum diameter are necessary.*

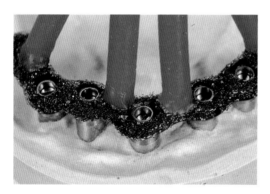

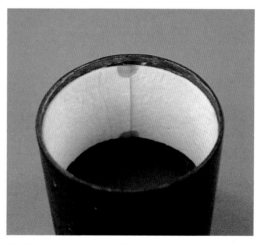

Fig 7-13 c *Formers are directed so that metal will be introduced into the pattern chamber at positions between gold cylinders.*

Fig 7-14 *Ring liner with a 2 mm ring exposure space for direct investment to ring contact.*

material can become detached during investing. Sprues aimed at gold cylinders, encourages their displacement on metal entry and increases the possibility of turbulence porosity. Care should also be taken that the attachment of the formers does not prevent screwdriver removal of the gold screws (Figs 7-13 a–c). If the pattern must be made larger than that de-scribed because of additional implants, then more sprue formers than this will be required.

The free ends of the sprues are finally organised into an apex, the underside of which has a smoothly rounded shape. This precaution avoids investment rough-ness and possible fracture at this point. The whole is then left undisturbed for 16

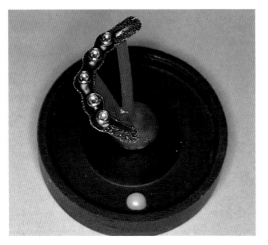

Fig 7-15 a *Pattern mounted on a crucible former. Note position of wax bead on the crucible former.*

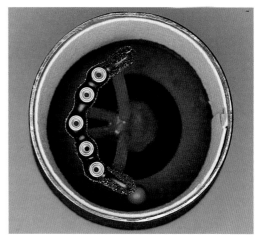

Fig 7-15 b *The curve of the pattern should be brought to an even distance with the side of the ring.*

hours (overnight) or longer before continuing.

RING LINING

The casting ring is prepared with one layer of Kaoliner ceramic fibre ring lining material (g). This material has been found to be adequately compressible for the expansion of the recommended investments used. The liner is positioned so that a gap of 2–3 mm exists at the top (pattern position) of the ring with a 1–2 mm overlap of the cut edges. The gap allows investment to contact the ring sides for greater security. The liner is secured to the ring with a few drops of molten wax placed on the joint line (Fig 7-14).

Most cellulose paper materials are less suitable liners in that they have been found to allow gypsum–bonded investment moulds to crack at casting temperature.

MOULD ORIENTATION MARKER FOR CENTRIFUGAL CASTING

A wax bead attached to the crucible former in a standardised position forms a pattern chamber position indicator. In reaction to the anti–clockwise direction of centrifugal casting arm rotation, molten metal flows into the mould, favouring the 'trailing edge' of arm rotation. When sprues are aligned to this trailing edge, metal will then travel more directly into them and the waiting pattern chamber beyond. The bead forms a depression on the surface of the mould which aids its positioning in the waiting casting machine.

PATTERN PREPARATION

After an overnight or longer interval of pattern strain relief the screws retaining the pattern are removed, whilst momentarily retaining one in a cantilever implant as a final verification of a perfect fit. The completed pattern and sprue system is then mounted on the crucible former, so that the gold cylinders are brought to an uppermost position. A correct orientation brings the pattern to an even space with the ring sides, with no pattern part closer than 10 mm to the sides of the ring liner and 6 mm to the open ring end (Figs 7-15 a and b).

INVESTMENTS

Whip Mix Cristobalite and Beauty–Cast (f), and Kerr Cristobalite (c) gypsum–bonded investments have been found to give accurate expansion results with Stabilor G alloy. Beauty–Cast is intended to be used in either a hygroscopic expansion or preferred thermal expansion mode.

All investments deteriorate when exposed to the atmosphere. For this reason materials supplied in sealed, pre–weighed packets are preferred. *It is mandatory that the investment manufacturers recommended powder/water ratio's and mixing times are accurately followed.*

INVESTING AND MOULD HEATING

Because patterns can distort from ambient temperature variations, investing should take place with the minimum delay after removal from the master cast. The opportunity for distortion from this cause is further reduced when investing materials are stored and used at the same laboratory temperature. The use of room temperature water for mixing is particularly recommended.

The lined ring is completely submerged in water and left to drain, while the pattern and sprue formers are treated with a surface tension reducing liquid. Jelenko Wax Pattern Cleaner has the advantage of a spray delivery which reaches otherwise inaccessible pattern parts (h). The treated pattern is allowed to dry or, alternatively, is gently blown dry before investing. This is important. Patterns invested wet have an increased surface roughness after casting. Three hundred grams of investment powder will be necessary to fill the recommended casting ring.

Investments are mechanically mixed under vacuum, as directed by the manufacturer. After releasing the vacuum, the investment is poured steadily into a vibrating casting ring under normal atmospheric pressure. Pouring takes place at a position in the ring, remote from the pattern. Investment material will be seen to flow into, and emerge through, each gold cylinder before filling the ring with a slight excess. The instant the mould is completely filled vibration is stopped (Figs 7-16 a–c).

Investments set with a smooth glazed surface. The increased density of this layer at the open ring end increases back pressure resistance and retards metal entry into the mould. This is avoided by cutting away set excess investment flush with the ring end, to reveal its full internal porosity.

Whip Mix and Kerr recommend a minimum investment setting time of 30 minutes before beginning burn–out [mould heating]. Research has shown that when the setting time of these materials is increased to 60 minutes, room temperature and casting temperature strengths are substantially increased.[1] Also shown, is that moisture contained within recently set

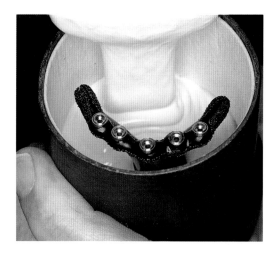
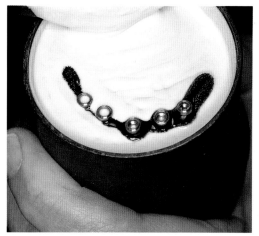
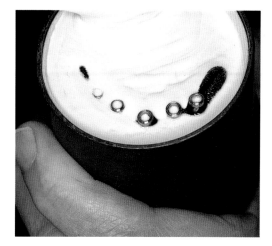

Fig 7-16 a–c   *Vacuum mixed investment is poured into the ring under vibration, at a position remote from the pattern. Investment is seen to emerge and flow through the cylinders, pouring continues until the ring is filled to a slight excess.*

investment, acts as a necessary 'heat buffer', which reduces thermal shock mould cracking during heating. As furnace temperature increases, the rise in internal mould temperature is initially delayed by boiling evaporation of the residual moisture. As this is reduced, mould temperature gradually increases, eventually to follow that of increasing furnace temperature and mould cracking is avoided. Mould heating, therefore, should begin shortly after a 60 minutes setting time or,

alternatively, the mould should be kept in a sealed moisture retaining container until convenient.

After the crucible former has been removed, surface investment debris are removed from the crucible by rinsing the entire mould in water. The mould is then placed, sprue channels downwards, in a room temperature furnace and heated to 690 °C. Because of a delay in the centre of the mould reaching the final furnace temperature, the mould is heat—soaked at

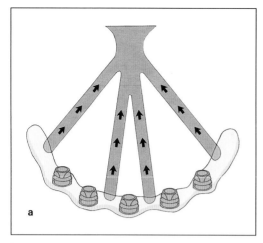 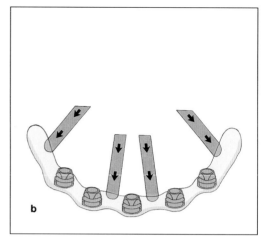

Fig 7-17 *Connected sprues contract together to distort the framework (a). Unconnected sprues can contract or otherwise alter their dimensions as they wish, without affecting the framework (b).*

690 °C for 30–40 minutes before casting. Heat–soak times much in excess of 45–50 minutes encourage mould cracking.

AMOUNT OF CASTING METAL REQUIRED

When castings solidify from their molten state they contract. The sprue system also contracts and distorts the casting to which it is attached (Fig 7-17 a). Worse than this, when sprues are connected by subsidiary runners, a secondary complex of metal may be formed which has an equal, if not greater, volume than that of the framework. Distortion resulting from this will then be correspondingly greater.

This sprue induced misfitting is entirely avoided by not allowing the cast sprues to join with each other or form a button of excess metal. When cast sprues do not connect in this way the individually separate 'sprue rods' formed can then independently contract without effect on the framework to which they are attached. This is an important factor in casting accuracy (Fig 7-17 b).

The smaller amount of metal required by this method has the added advantage of economy and the removed diminutive sprues form a smaller proportion of 'used' metal for the next casting. The latter tending to preserve the composition and mechanical properties of the re–cast alloy. Metal estimation is not difficult. Finished Stabilor G frameworks usually weigh between 10 gm and 15 gm, complete with incorporated gold cylinders. Cast sprues of 4 mm diameter and 30 mm in length weigh approximately 5 gm each. Assuming that every framework will weigh 15 gm and each of the 4 sprues need only be approximately half full, then a total weight of 25 gm of Stabilor G alloy should safely suffice. If wider sprues are used then correspondingly more metal will be required.

This alloy weight estimation applies

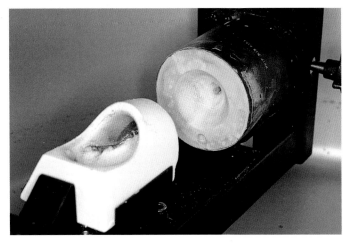
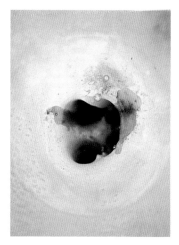

Fig 7-18 (left)   *Mould orientation marker indicates the position of the mould in the casting machine to most efficiently receive the melt.*

Fig 7-18 b (right)   *Appearance of correctly cast mould with open sprues and absence of excess button.*

only to metals with specific gravities of between 14 and 15 g/cm³.

If an excess of metal is inadvertently used and sprue connection occurs, then providing that all other parts of the described technique have been followed and especially equal sprue former length, smaller frameworks will still have a satisfactory fit without corrective soldering.

PRE–CASTING MOULD COOLING

As moulds wait in the casting machine to be cast they cool. They also contract and this occurs at a greater and faster rate than the expansion which occurred during heating. Also, moulds do not cool uniformly. Outer mould parts cool first, this then produces a temperature difference compared with its inner core material, a differential which distorts the mould.[1] This cooling interval is minimised by pre–heating (but not melting) the alloy prior to

mould removal from the furnace. The target mould cooling interval before casting should be less than 20 seconds. This seemingly brief interval is easily and safely achieved in practice. Using the mould depression marker as a guide, the heated ring is quickly and accurately placed in the casting machine to receive the melt (Fig 7-18 a).

After casting, each sprue orifice should be open and it may not be possible to see metal in them; when this proven method is first tried this appearance can be disconcerting (Fig 7-18 b).

STRENGTHENING HEAT TREATMENT

The cast mould is removed from the casting machine and placed on a heat resistant surface to cool undisturbed and unassisted to room temperature.

It must be finally possible to hold the air cooled mould with bare hands before re-

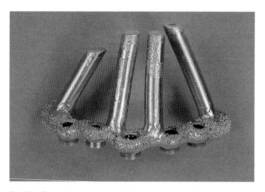 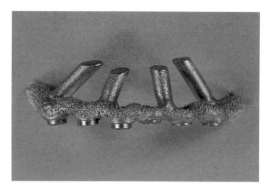

Fig 7-19 a + b *As—cast frameworks showing unconnected sprues.*

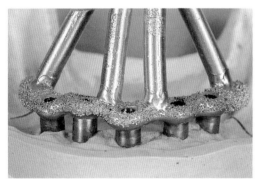 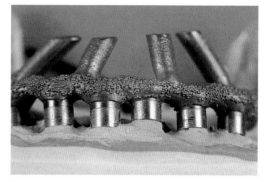

Fig 7-19 c + d *The overall fit of frameworks with only one gold screw tightened to place in a cantilever replica.*

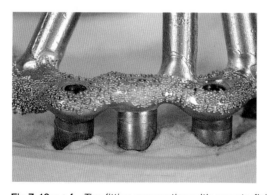 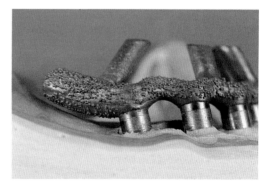

Fig 7-19 e + f *The fitting connection with remote fixing screws.*

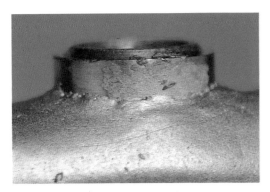

Fig 7-20 a *Thin flash of cast metal attached to the side of a gold cylinder.*

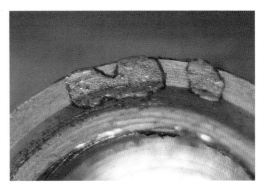

Fig 7-20 b *The fitting surface of a cylinder spoiled by attached cast metal.*

moving the casting. This cooling interval will take approximately 45 minutes. *Do not accelerate or delay the rate of mould cooling.*

The obvious reason for selecting high strength type 4 alloys is their use in situations of high stress. If the manufacturers recommended heat treatment strengthening is not performed, type 4 mechanical properties will not be obtained. For this reason, and despite investment manufacturers clear instructions to the contrary, moulds containing Stabilor G castings must not be cooled in water. When this alloy is slow cooled to room temperature it automatically acquires its optimum mechanical strength properties without further heat treatment. Because of this feature, it is not necessary to return frameworks to the furnace for heat treatment strengthening, a process which carries some risk of distorting large castings.

Only after cooling to room temperature is the mould submerged in water, a precaution which reduces the production of investment dust during the removal of the casting from the mould. The inhalation of investment dust is injurious to health.

THE FIT OF FRAMEWORKS

Recovered castings are brushed clean in water and dried before pickling. The sprues should be separate and will be of varying length depending on the speed of casting arm rotation at the moment of alloy solidification (Figs 7-19 a and b). Fitting accuracy to the master cast is at first tested with finger pressure, before using one screw in either of the cantilever abutment replicas. The framework should have an accurate horizontal and perpendicular fit under ×20 magnification. An identical fit should apply wherever a single screw may be tightened to place. Providing that the recommended pattern dimensions and sprue former diameters are used, sprues need only be 10 mm long to prevent contraction porosity (Figs 7-19 c–f).

If the framework fails to fit, then the fitting surfaces of the gold cylinders should be individually examined under the microscope for thermal damage and the abutment replicas for mechanical damage or attached debris. Cast metal can flow down the sides of cylinders and

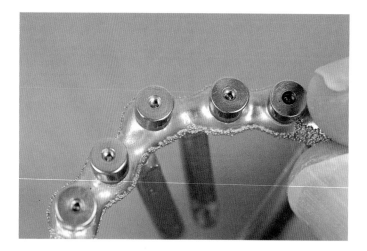

Fig 7-21 a *Protective polishing caps fitted to gold cylinders.*

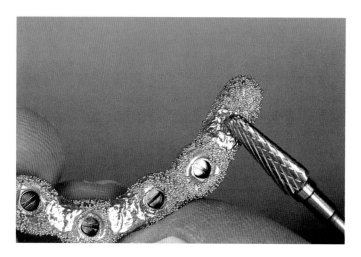

Fig 7-21 b *Re-shaping sprue attachment areas.*

onto the fitting surfaces of cylinders to spoil their fitting (Figs 7-20 a and b); a fault caused by cylinder movement in the pattern chamber due to wax covering the upper rim surface of the cylinder, wax residues left on the skirt of the cylinder, sprue formers directed at cylinders or over—expanded moulds.

If accurate abutment replicas have been used, misfitting errors will be easily seen and no amount of finger pressure or other persuasion will remove them.

FRAMEWORK FINISHING

The machined fitting surfaces of gold cylinders are highly vulnerable to damage during required framework polishing processes. Stainless steel Protection Caps (i) screw fitted to the cylinders prevent this damage and are quite essential (Fig 7-21 a). The caps have a slightly larger diameter than the cylinders and so extend to overlap for additional protection. Some texts recommend the use of cut—down

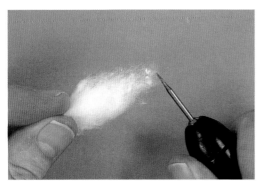

Fig 7-22 a *Cotton wool about to be caught by a rotating fissure bur.*

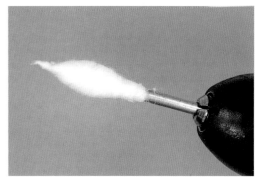

Fig 7-22 b *Compacted material automatically tightened round the bur to form a polishing bud.*

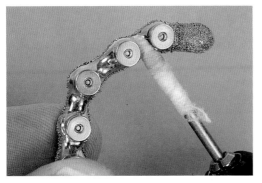

Fig 7-22 c *When impregnated with polishing compound the bud can reach and polish in otherwise inaccessible places.*

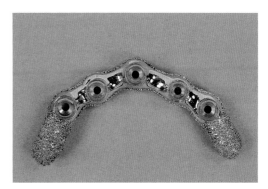

Fig 7-22 d *Finished framework.*

abutment replicas for this work, however, these are much inferior.

The sprues are removed and the area of their attachment ground to the original contour (Fig 7-21 b). Abrasive rubber wheels, felt, cotton and wool polishing mops used with Tripoli and rouge will provide exposed framework parts with a high polish. Sometimes the space existing between cylinders is inaccessibly small. Laterally reduced wheels and mops will generally deal with this. The polishing bud is also useful. A rotating fissure bur will unfailingly collect and wind a small piece

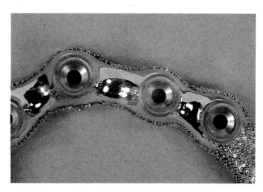

Fig 7-22 e *Detail showing bead retention finishing with a neat edge and undamaged gold cylinders.*

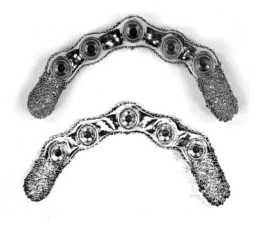

Fig 7-23 a *A photocopy of the framework provides a satisfactory record of work.*

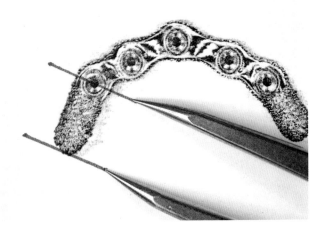

Fig 7-23 b *The image accurately records several important dimensions.*

of cotton wool around itself to make an efficient polisher. When used with Tripoli or other polishing compound, it will efficiently provide a high polish in even the most inaccessible areas (Figs 7-22 a–e). A final ultrasonic or pressure steam cleaning completes this work.

The weight of alloy used to cast the illustrated framework and attached sprues complete was approximately 25.00 gm. The unpolished framework with contained gold cylinders weighed 14.50 gm and removed sprues 12.50 gm. Since 4 mm gold cylinders each weigh 0.40 gm, the weight of alloy required to make the framework was 12.50 gm. Three millimetre high gold cylinders each weigh 0.30 gm.

RECORDING FRAMEWORK DIMENSIONS

An accurate and inexpensive record of

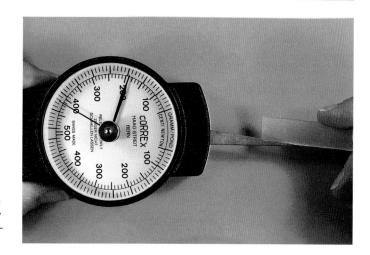

Fig 7-24 a *A strip of modelling wax 13 mm wide at approximately 20°C can exert a maximum pressure of approximately 200 gm.*

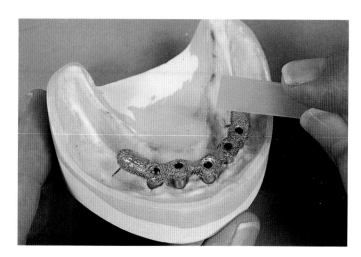

Fig 7-24 b *Testing the fit of a framework by pressure from a wax strip.*

frameworks is made by photocopying them. Although mainly a profile image, this clearly shows the principal dimensions, including cantilever length upon which can be superimposed the position of occlusal tables and other features as required (Figs 7-23 a and b). Such information is essential if long–term success rates of implants and prostheses are to be objectively audited.

FINAL FITTING INSPECTION

It sometimes occurs that the very slightest 'shadow' or suspicion of a vertical discrepancy exists between a gold cylinder and abutment replica, remote from the single test screw, and slight pressure from a finger tip appears to close it. Such is the error magnification of the Sheffield test, that this may be due to minute traces of wax or polishing debris on one or more replicas or gold cylinders. These parts

127

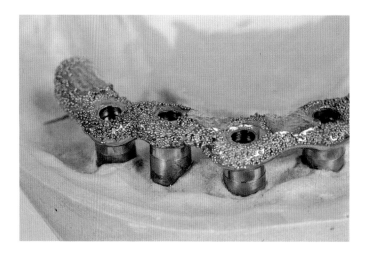

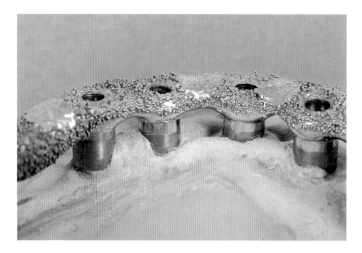

Fig 7-25 a + b   *Finished framework ready for trial in the mouth.*

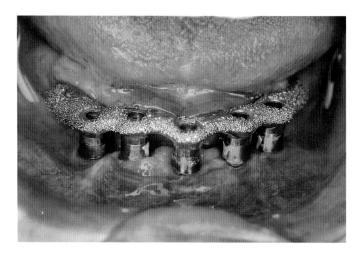

Fig 7-26   *Fit of framework in the mouth with one screw in a cantilever implant.*

should be scrupulously steam cleaned before test fitting.

In these cases, a satisfactory fit may be confirmed by the following test. It can be shown that the edge of a 13 mm wide strip of modelling wax at a room temperature of approximately 20 °C can exert a force of about 200 gm before buckling.

If a suspected fitting discrepancy can be closed by pressure from this strip of wax, then the fit is satisfactory without further attention (Figs 7-24 a and b).

FRAMEWORK TRY—IN AND JAW REGISTRATION

The finished framework is delivered for trial in the mouth with one slave gold screw or guide pin in place. By this presentation the dentist is more able to assess the quality of work, before trial in the mouth (Figs 7-25 a and b).

The same fitting test is repeated in the mouth, except that a new gold screw is used (Fig 7-26). The clinician may also wish to place a complete set of new screws for a final verification that all is satisfactory. This work is quickly done and the opportunity may be taken to register the jaw relation at the same visit.

Pre—formed wax rims are conveniently softened in hot water and attached to the framework using hard wax. Many dentists prefer the convenience of a single short guide pin or gold screw in an anterior implant, to retain the framework/registration rim during the registration of jaw relationships.

REFERENCE

1. White G E. The resistance of selected dental casting investments to casting stresses. PhD thesis. Department of Restorative Dentistry, University of Sheffield. 1987.

CHAPTER 7: MATERIALS AND EQUIPMENT

Manufacturer	UK Suppliers

(a) Special Tray resin
De Trey Division
Dentsply Limited
Hamm Moor Lane
Addlestone
Weybridge
KT15 2SE

(b) Dura Lay resin
Reliance Dental Manufacturing Co	Associated Dental Products Ltd
Worth	Kemdent Works
Illinois	Purton
USA	Swindon
	FN5 9HT

(c) Inlay casting wax
Cristobalite investment
Kerr Manufacturing Co	Kerr (UK) Limited
Romulus	27 Coningsby Road
Michigan	Bretton
USA	Peterborough
	PE3 8SB

(d) Ash No. 5 wax carving instrument
Ash Instruments Division
Dentsply Limited
Hamm Moor Lane
Addlestone
Weybridge
KT15 2SE

(e) Veneer—Lock beads
George Taub Products and	Dentomax Limited
Fusion Co Inc	Carr House
277 New York Ave	Carrbottom Road
Jersey City	Bradford
NJ 07307	BD5 9BJ
USA	

Manufacturer	UK Suppliers
(f) Casting ring and crucible former **Cristobalite and Beauty Cast Investments** Whip Mix Corporation 361 Framlington Avenue PO Box 17183 Louisville Kentucky 40217 USA	Skillbond Limited Dudley House Gordon Road High Wycombe HP 13 6 EL
(g) Kaoliner ring liner Dentsply International Inc York PA 17405 USA	Dentsply Limited Hamm Moor Lane Addlestone Weybridge KT15 2SE
(h) Jelenko Wax Pattern Cleaner Pennwalt Jelenko 99 Business Park Drive Armonk NY USA	Skillbond Limited Dudley House Gordon Road High Wycombe HP13 6 EL
(i) Polishing Protection Caps Nobelpharma AB Box 5190 S-402 26 Gothenburg Sweden	Nobelpharma UK Ltd Nobel House Packet Boat Lane Uxbridge UB8 2GH

Chapter Eight

Setting—up and Finishing Fixed Complete Prostheses

Casts and registration blocks are mounted on either average condylar movement or adjustable condylar path articulators. Condylator machines have been found to be accurate and convenient when used with implant supported prostheses (a). This articulators automatic imprinting of its serial number onto work also proves useful (Figs 8-1a and b). Items which are identified in this way allow for a mixture of current work and archived material from different patients to be accurately returned to the original articulator.

Implant supported prostheses are able to exert a biting force closely equivalent, if not identical, to the dentate state.[1] This fact has important implications for the design

of opposing prostheses. For example, when a patient with an implant supported mandibular prosthesis is also edentulous in the opposing jaw, the situation of natural lower teeth opposing a complete upper denture is almost replicated. An important difference, however, is that the position and occlusion of all the teeth is under the control of the prosthodontist and the technician.

As osseointegrated implants lack a periodontium, the use of resin teeth has been recommended to provide certain shock absorbing qualities.[2] Good quality resin teeth also have adequate wear resisting properties and can easily be provided with screw access holes, the latter being an important advantage. Porcelain

Fig 8-1 a   *Condylator articulator serial number.*

Fig 8-1 b   *Articulator number reproduced in plaster—work.*

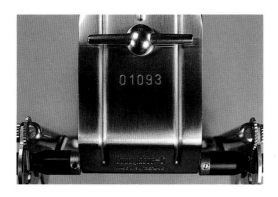

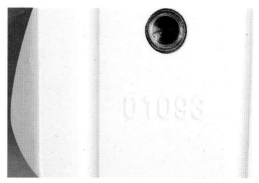

teeth are impossibly difficult to alter in this respect.

An important consideration when short fixtures and poor, or grafted bone conditions exist is the need to reduce occlusal stress on these parts for a period following confirmed osseointegration. Although cantilevers of a final length may have been provided, a novice tooth set—up, consisting of fewer and/or narrower artificial teeth, will temporarily reduce occlusal stress. After a period of about 12–18 months, the patient will return to have this altered and the final number and/or size of teeth positioned. Alternatively, an intermediate prosthesis may have been worn for a sufficient post—osseointegration bone remodelling interval, which makes this unnecessary (Chapter 4).

Trial Dentures

After the master casts have been made there are two methods in which to progress to the jaw registration and prosthesis try—in stages.

Method 1

When an intermediate prosthesis is worn, or the space between the residual ridges is large and the implants are in helpful positions, the framework can be made before the teeth are set—up.

A wax occlusal rim is conveniently attached to the framework at the time of its test fitting and a registration of jaw relation made with the framework connected to the implants. Frameworks of the recommended design are conveniently small so do not usually interfere with the future positions of the teeth.

Advantages of method 1

1. Regardless of bone resorption, the implant retained rim is stable during jaw registration.
2. The positions of unhelpfully sited implants and their screw access holes are revealed during setting-up and the best compromise tooth appearance obtained for consideration at the first try—in.
3. Fewer treatment visits for the patient.

Disadvantages

1. The framework may be made without knowing the existence of abnormal jaw and/or tooth relationships.
2. The space between the residual ridges may be small, causing gross tooth interferences with the framework which could have been avoided by the use of shorter gold cylinders and/or altered framework shape.

Setting—up the teeth

The master casts and occlusal rims are mounted onto the articulator using a face—bow record or statistically average position.

Tapered model sides form an accurate socket in the articulating plaster for the return of casts and dentures after processing (Fig 8-2).

The upper incisor and canine teeth are set first to appearance criteria, followed by sufficient upper posterior teeth having an anterior—posterior dimension equal to the given cantilever length. If the upper residual ridge has been assessed as good, then either one or two premolars and a molar tooth will be set on each side, depending on cantilever length and applying horizontal jaw relationship. Alter-

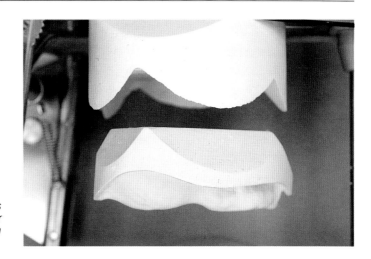

Fig 8-2 *Tapered model sides produce an accurate master cast/denture remount socket in the articulating plaster.*

natively, if the maxillary foundations are poor, then these teeth are narrowed or the molar is discarded and only premolar teeth are used. This smaller novice occlusal table acts to reduce the size of masticatory load transmitted to the underlying bone (Fig 8-3 a).

Lower posterior teeth are now set with regard to the cantilever length and the teeth already placed on the upper denture. Although the mandibular teeth will correctly intercuspate, their number may not numerically match those set in the upper. If a less than ideal number and length of fixtures have been installed, and/or the bone is of poor quality, the obtaining occlusal table may consist of only two upper and two lower posterior teeth in occlusion on each side (Figs 8-3 b and c). This potentially unstable upper denture situation is improved by substituting upper premolar teeth for upper canine teeth[3] (Fig 8-3 d and e).

The lower canine teeth now occlude in

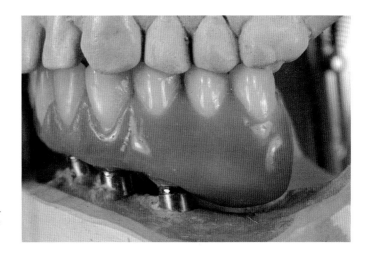

Fig 8-3 a *Three lower premolar teeth providing a novice reduced occlusal table.*

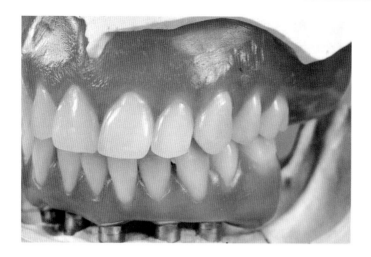

Fig 8-3 b *Completed set—up ready for trial in the mouth.*

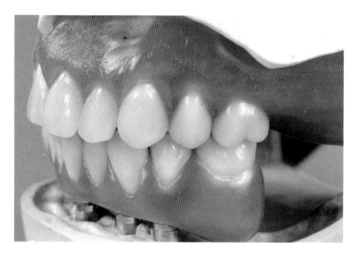

Fig 8-3 c *Carefully short cantilevers may mean that there are only two upper and two lower posterior teeth in occlusion.*

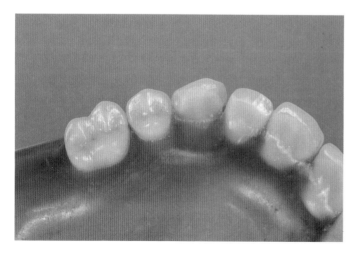

Fig 8-3 d *Size of occlusal table when only two posterior teeth can be placed.*

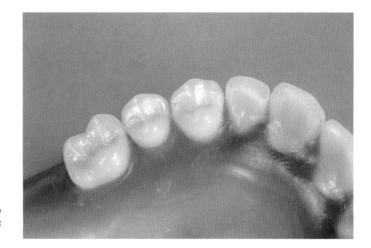

Fig 8-3 e *Size of occlusal table when an upper premolar tooth is substituted for the upper canine.*

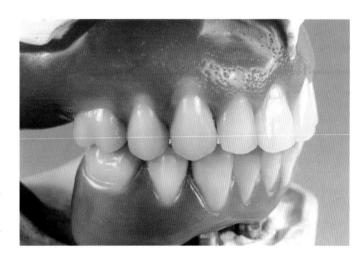

Fig 8-3 f *The upper canine/premolar substitution brings three teeth into occlusion without increasing the length of the canti-levers.*

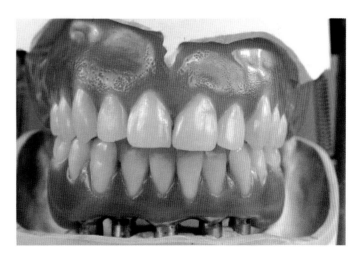

Fig 8-3 g *The appearance of premolar–canines can deceive the eye to give a good appearance.*

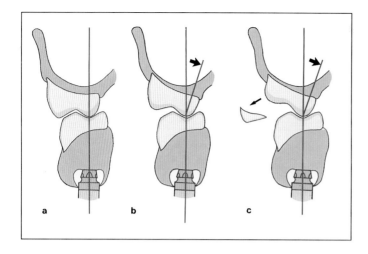

Fig 8-4   *When the maxillary ridge is well formed the posterior teeth maximally intercuspate (a). When the maxillary ridge is unsatisfactory the upper teeth are tilted to remove buccal cusps from contact with the lower teeth (b). When the upper ridge is very poor the posterior teeth are tilted and the buccal cusps removed by grinding (c).*

the central fossae of the premolar substitutes, so increasing the size of occlusal table in an anterior direction. The number of teeth in occlusion is thereby increased without extension of the cantilevers. This mechanically advantageous device is not immediately obvious (Figs 8-3 f and g). Whatever the implant and bone foundations, the most posteriorly set lower tooth will not extend beyond the end of a 13 mm cantilever. Novice occlusions will be short of this measure.

When the maxillary residual ridge forms a satisfactory foundation the teeth are set to maximally intercuspate (Fig 8-4 a). When this ridge is less than well provided, the upper posterior teeth are tilted and/or ground to remove their buccal cusps from contact with the lower teeth, while preserving palatal cusp contacts (Fig 8-4 b). This has two advantages, denture displacing buccal cusp pressures are reduced and forces of mastication directed more centrally over the maxillary ridge crest (Fig 8-4 c).[4]

Method 2

Using this method setting—up precedes framework construction. Jaw registration and trial dentures are made on resin bases which rest over plastic healing cap protected implants and on the mucosa (Figs 8-5 a and b). The lower trial prosthesis resembles an overdenture without connection to the implants, with the lower posterior teeth restricted to a space which duplicates future cantilever length.

The wax trial denture is tested in the mouth without attachment to the implants. This approach is particularly useful when the inter—ridge distance is small and there are unhelpful jaw, tooth and fixture relationships. After the denture has been successfully tested, a framework is then made to carry the teeth in their now established positions.

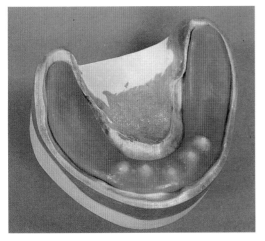

Fig 8-5 a *Self—curing resin base covering the healing caps.*

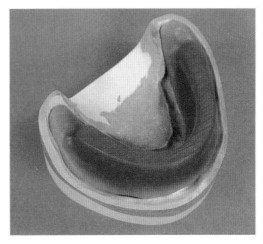

Fig 8-5 b *Completed occlusal rim.*

Advantages of method 2

1. The appearance of the teeth and their occlusion can be established before the framework is made.
2. Because fixing screws are not used, the occlusal rims and trial denture are easily inserted and removed from the mouth for chairside adjustments.
3. The patient may take the trial dentures away for assessment at home.

Disadvantages

1. The future position of gold screw access holes and framework parts cannot be assessed, so tooth positions may be approved which are not technically possible.
2. The registration of jaw relationships and the try—in are assessed on bases which may rest on unfavourable ridges and moveable mucosa.
3. Additional treatment visits are necessary.

Setting—up the teeth

The design cantilever lengths are marked on the sides of the cast and the dentures set—up for appearance and function without regard to implant positions (Fig 8-6 a). The last upper and lower posterior tooth on each side of the jaw will not be set beyond the pencil mark showing future cantilever length (Fig 8-6 b). The remaining teeth are set to the principals described in Method 1.

When the dentures have been approved in the mouth, the position of the lower teeth is recorded by means of an imprint key made in Lab Putty (b). The framework is now made and the teeth from the trial denture re—set on the framework using the key.

As from this stage methods 1 and 2 follow the same pattern.

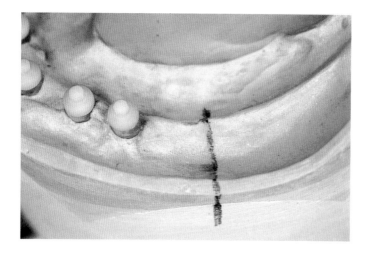

Fig 8-6 a *Pencil mark indicating the end of the future 13 mm long framework cantilever.*

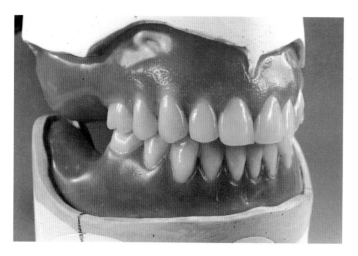

Fig 8-6 b *Completed trial dentures with canine/premolar substitution. Teeth set for appearance and function without regard to implant position or screw access holes.*

SCREW ACCESS HOLES

Favourably installed implants will be on or near the crest of the residual ridges so beneath the occlusal surfaces of the artificial posterior teeth. Functional loads arriving on these teeth will then be transmitted to bone along the long axis of the implant which is mechanically efficient. The only disadvantage in this arrangement is that the gold screw access holes will emerge through the teeth. These 2.4 mm diameter access holes and their position form a fixed factor around which dental technology must do what it can to provide the best tooth appearance and adequately intact occlusal surfaces.

When setting—up is completed it is then easy to see where the screws will emerge and which teeth will require screw access perforation.

Each necessary tooth is removed in turn and a guide pin placed in lieu of a gold screw. The position of a small pilot

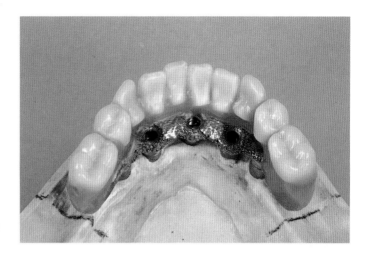

Fig 8-7 a *Resin teeth set onto framework.*

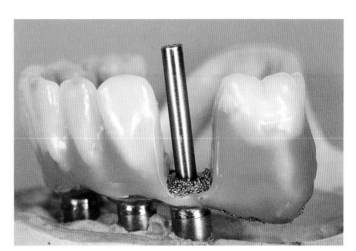

Fig 8-7 b *Guide pin indicating the required position of screw access hole in the removed tooth.*

hole is then checked before enlargement with larger burrs, until the guide pin comfortably protrudes through the tooth (Figs 8-7 a–d). The manufactured pin lengths of 10, 15 and 20 mm are not always convenient: too short and the slotted head is buried beneath the surface of the tooth or denture base, too long and the head projects well beyond the denture. Pins may be shortened as necessary and new screwdriver slots cut with a disc. A selection of altered guide pins is very useful.

When necessary it is usually possible to slightly adjust the positions of individual teeth to contain holes within occlusal surfaces or neatly between teeth. If despite this care an access hole emerges through a labial or buccal tooth surface, then let it. The offending hole can be dealt with by the dentist using tooth coloured filling material after installing the denture.

With all guide pins in position, the trial denture is waxed and shaped, remembering that the patient will not be able to re-

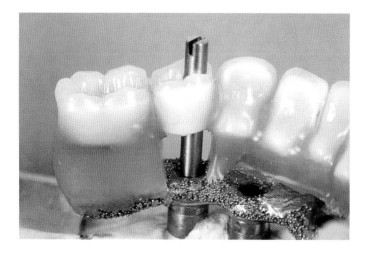

Fig 8-7 c   *Perforated tooth returned to position.*

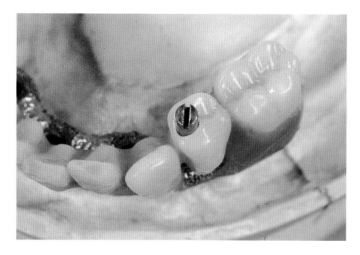

Fig 8-7 d   *Head of pin correctly protruding through tooth.*

move the prosthesis for cleaning (Figs 8-8 a–c and Fig 12-1 b). When novice occlusions are provided on frameworks which have a final cantilever length, unused cantilever parts will also need a thin covering of wax.

It is a good idea to test the cleaning access of trial prostheses using the small brushes which will be used by the patient, not forgetting the increased difficulty of brush access in the rear of the mouth.

When bone resorption is advanced, the position of the correctly restored occlusal plane can be a startlingly large distance from a resorbed residual ridge. A distance of 2 cm is not unusual (Fig 8-9).

TRY—IN OF DENTURES AND FINISHING

As well as the more usual assessments, the dentist will also check cleaning access to the abutments and especially

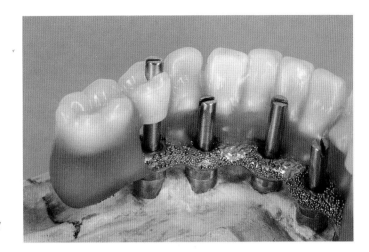

Fig 8-8 a *Guide pins of altered length screwed to position.*

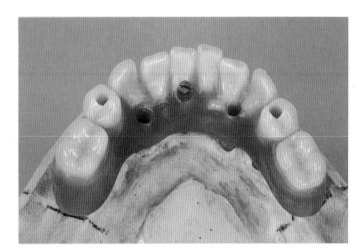

Fig 8-8 b *Completed trial denture retained with one guide pin.*

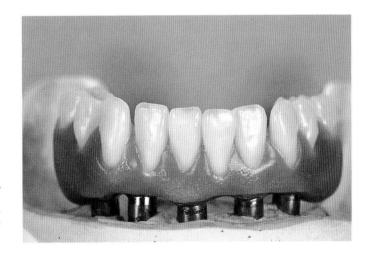

Fig 8-8 c *Waxed denture ready for trial in the mouth. Note absence of visible metalwork which is usual with Sheffield frameworks.*

143

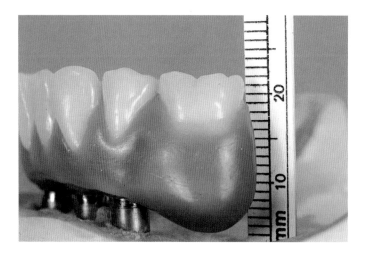

Fig 8-9 *A correctly restored occlusal vertical height can result in a large prosthesis. Note rounded form of under cantilever parts to provide easy cleaning access.*

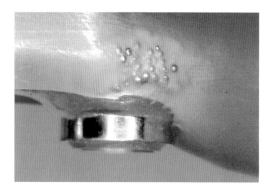

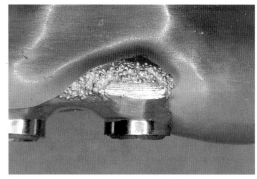

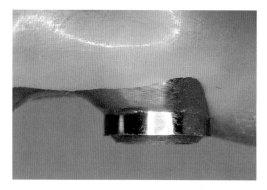

Fig 8-10 a (above left) *Wax brought to a thin edge which almost exposes the framework beneath.*

Fig 8-10 b (above right) *Retention beads ground away and a wax/resin finishing gutter cut into the framework with a disc.*

Fig 8-10 c *Re—waxed prosthesis with an adequate thickness of wax covering the framework.*

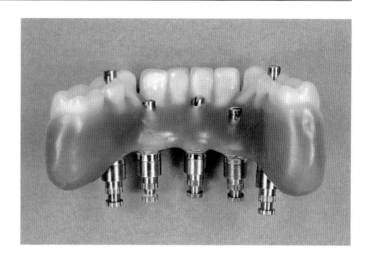

Fig 8-11 a *Abutment replicas held in place with cut–down guide pins.*

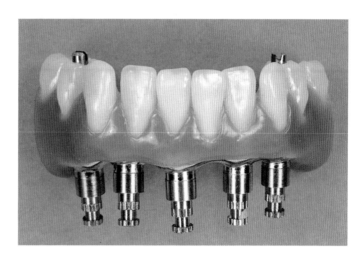

Fig 8-11 b *Denture ready for investing and processing. The wax stippling shown in Fig 8-8 c has been removed by flaming.*

under cantilever parts. Any chairside adjustments of the wax and teeth are made good and attention given to achieving a neat wax to framework junction finish. Larger revisions of tooth position can sometimes bring new wax to delicately thin edges in some framework parts and especially adjacent to gold cylinders. When this occurs the bead retention is ground away and individually separate and circumspect gutters cut using small carborundum discs (Figs 8-10 a–c).

PROCESSING

It is not necessary to process the implant denture on its master cast. Used abutment replicas may alternatively be connected to the gold cylinders using guide pins. When invested in a processing flask the replicas will be held in the investing plaster so taking the place of the master cast. Guide pins must not project more than 2–3 mm beyond the surface of the denture (Figs 8-11 a and b). Any wax

145

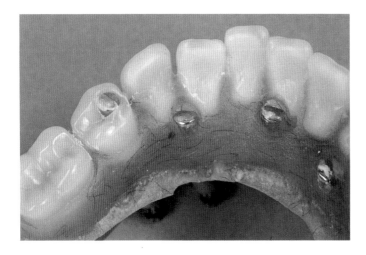

Fig 8-12 a *Polymerised denture with resin covering the screw-driver slots in the guide pins.*

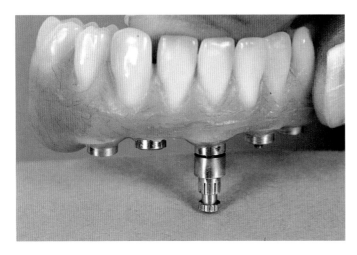

Fig 8-12 b *Pressure on a partly unscrewed replica will usually loosen the guide pin.*

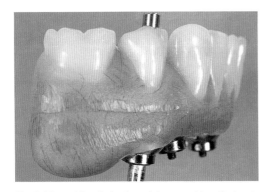

Fig 8-12 c *Mandrel placed in a gold cylinder in contact with the threaded end of a guide pin.*

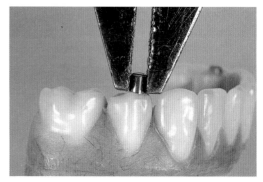

Fig 8-12 d *Pliers removing a loosened guide pin with a twisting pull.*

stippling provided for assessment at the try–in is now removed by flaming to produce a smooth surface. This will be replaced by different means at a later stage.

The denture is processed following complete denture practice. The framework and abutment replicas will be contained in one flask half, with the teeth in the other. After wax removal and application of mould sealant, the mould is packed with heat–cured denture base resin and polymerised according to the manufacturers instructions. Framework opaquing concealment will almost certainly not be necessary, provided that translucent denture base resin is not used.

After polymerisation the flask is allowed to slowly cool to room temperature. This minimises occlusal disturbances of the teeth, especially in thick prostheses. Auto-polymerising resin may also be used without flasking, but these materials may be less wear resistant.

Grinding–in the occlusion

After recovery from the flask, the abutment replicas are unscrewed from the denture framework. Resin flash will now fill the screwdriver slots in the guide pins, this must be removed with a hot knife before attempting pin withdrawl. Sometimes pins stubbornly resist removal. A firm tap on their threaded end from a mandrel placed carefully through the gold cylinder will loosen them. Pressure on the end of a partly unscrewed replica is also effective (Fig 8-12 a–c). Loosened pins are finally extracted using parallel opening pliers and a twisting pull (Fig 8-12 d). The denture can now be returned to its master cast and secured there with one or more

slave gold screws. Guide pins are now a tight fit, so are less convenient.

While still on its master cast, the upper prosthesis is returned to its articulator mounting socket and secured there using cyanoacrylate cement. This accurate denture remount procedure allows for an essential grinding–in removal of unavoidable processing errors and refinement of occlusal balance.[4,5]

Having first removed tooth contact prematuraties in centric occlusion by grinding, the articulator is then moved to simulate a complete envelope of border and inter-border mandibular movement. Using disclosing ribbon or thin articulating paper, identified tooth interferences are removed as they are found, until smooth gliding tooth contacts are achieved. The obtained occlusal balance is then refined using fine carborundum grinding paste between the teeth which merges the ground and un–ground areas into a single unified form. The articulator is moved in small 'rotary' movements during this work so that a combination of border and inter–border jaw movements are simulated. Through this work stability of the opposing conventional denture is improved and lateral forces acting on the prostheses and implants reduced.

Polishing

After protective polishing caps have been attached to the gold cylinders, resin adjacent to the screw access holes is shaped to the contour of the surrounding material and the resin/framework junction carefully organised. The resin gum–work may be bent bur stippled to resemble attached mucosa. Prepared by heating to a red heat in a Bunsen flame and bending with pliers before water quenching, small rose-

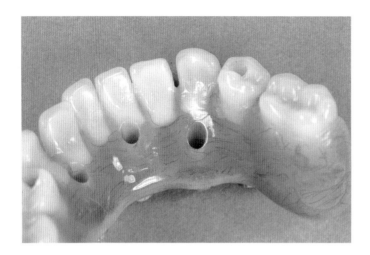

Fig 8-13 a   *Polished lingual denture parts with gold screw access holes in teeth and denture base.*

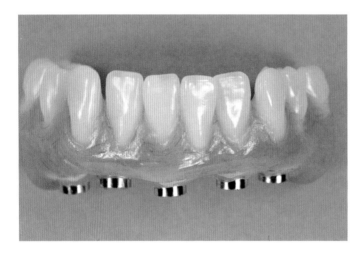

Fig 8-13 b   *Appearance of prosthesis. Note framework concealment and stippled attached gingiva.*

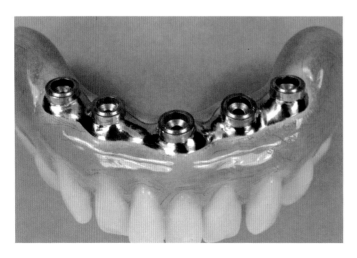

Fig 8-13 c   *Resin/framework junction. Note typically thick resin edges.*

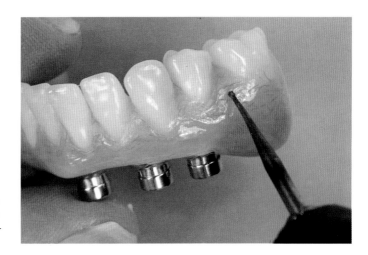

Fig 8-13 d *Revolving bent bur provides a realistic stippling effect which is easy for the patient to keep clean.*

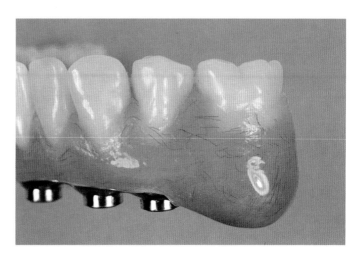

Fig 8-13 e *Cantilever under—parts have a rounded form and are highly polished.*

head burrs provide a realistic stippling effect which is easy for the patient to keep clean. The denture is then polished, again bearing in mind that the patient will not be able to remove the denture for cleaning (Figs 8-13 a–e).

FITTING THE PROSTHESIS

The prosthesis is installed in the mouth using new gold screws which are tight-ened by a torque wrench. The occlusion of the teeth is then checked before each screw access hole is filled with a temporary obturating material. The patient then experiences the first sensations of prosthesis security and restored biting power (Figs 8-14 a–d).

After some days, the patient returns for final screw pre—loading and a more durable access hole closure. The colour of this material differs slightly from that of the host tooth or denture resin. Through this

149

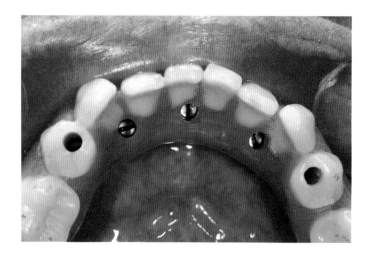

Fig 8-14 a *Prosthesis tightened in place in the mouth using gold screws in each implant.*

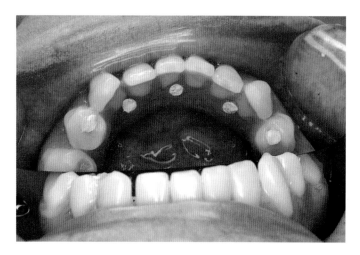

Fig 8-14 b *Installed lower prosthesis with temporarily closed screw access holes.*

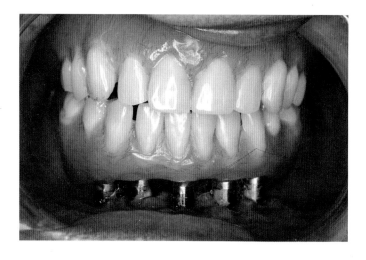

Fig 8-14 c *Appearance of complete upper and implant supported lower prosthesis.*

difference, screw positions are more easily revealed for future prosthesis removal.

ARCHIVING COMPLETED WORK ITEMS

During the years which follow, the prosthesis will need to be serviced and possibly repaired. With the virtual certainty of these events in mind, it is important to store laboratory prescription cards and other work items, such as models and articulator mountings for future use. Although treatment with implant supported prostheses offers the prospect of long—term treatment success, patients and their prostheses will surely return.

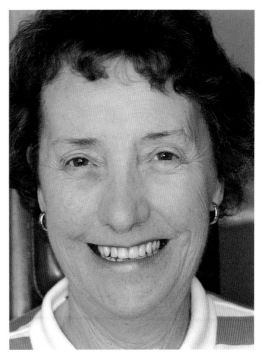

Fig 8-14 d *Patients appearance immediately after prosthesis installation.*

REFERENCES

1. Haraldson T, Carlsson G E, Ingervall B. Functional state, bite force and postural muscle activity in patients with osseointegrated oral implant bridges. *Acta Odontol Scand* 1979; 37: 195–206.

2. Skalak R. Biomechanical considerations in osseointegrated prostheses. *J Prosth Dent* 1983; 49: 843–848.

3. Gerber A. A short guide to improved complete prosthodontics. Complete dentures (1). Quintessence International Color Atlas. 1973. 27–32.

4. White G E. The Gerber articulator and system of full denture construction. Part 1. The Condylator articulator. *Dent Tech* 1973; 26: 12–20.

   Part 2 B. Setting—up the teeth and finishing the dentures. *Dent Tech* 1973; 26: 34–39.

5. Horn R, Stuck J. Zahnaufstellung in der Totalprothetik. Quintessenz Bibliothek, Berlin. 1980. (In German).

CHAPTER 8: MATERIALS AND EQUIPMENT

Manufacturer   UK Suppliers

(a) **Condylator articulators**
Condylator—Service
Bellariastraße 48
CH-8038 Zurich
Switzerland

(b) **Lab-Putty**
Coltène AG   Coltène (UK) Limited
Feldwiesenstraße 20   8a Teknol House
CH-9450 Altstätten   Victoria Road
Switzerland   Burgess Hill
                                  RH15 9LF

Chapter Nine
Overdentures

For many patients the seat of their dissatisfaction with conventional complete dentures is pain and instability in function and poor retention at other times. Problems which are made worse when the residual ridges are resorbed. If replacement dentures were connected to two or more implants in an otherwise mucosa supported denture, then the increased retention and security provided may be adequately sufficient. This principle forms the basis of overdenture design for both jaws, but is most commonly used in the mandible.

Although overdentures can provide a substantial increase in denture retention, there may not be an equal increase in functional stability. During mastication otherwise well retained overdentures can move to adversely stress their retention systems and damage this connection. Overdentures are frequently used where there is insufficient bone to support a fixed prosthesis. Consequent to this will be the use of shorter implants in the most resorbed residual ridges. Jemt et al.[1] reported that in the resorbed maxillary jaw there was a much increased failure rate of implants compared to fixed prostheses and that 22 % of the retaining clips fractured in the first year of use. Poor residual ridges imply denture movement in function. Whereas implant support can provide overdentures with a substantial increase in retention, it may not equally increase denture stability.

DENTURE INSTABILITY

Balanced occlusion of whatever refinement can not prevent functional denture instability. When conventional upper and lower complete dentures are apart and applying a closing force onto food, the teeth are also apart, so negating balance. The axiom 'entry food — exit balance' applies. When dentures are separated and under occlusal load it is the occlusal surfaces of the teeth relative to their underlying bone foundation which is relevant. Occlusal balance has no effect on tooth apart denture instability.

DESIGNING OVERDENTURES FOR FUNCTIONAL STABILITY

Full denture mechanics may be successfully applied to overdentures, in that posterior teeth should not be set over bone forming an angle to their occlusal surfaces. Despite the fact that posterior teeth may have been set to obtain efficient occlusal balance, occlusal loads arriving on the molar teeth can still be resolved in a manner which propels the denture in a

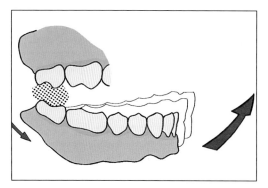

Fig 9-1 *Occlusal pressure on teeth set over inclined bone propels the denture in a forward direction.*

forward direction (Fig 9-1).[2] If the denture is retained by implants, then these and their mechanical connection with the denture will be laterally stressed by this movement. Implants and overdenture retention systems are not designed to resist horizontal stresses and are damaged by these loads.

TOOTH POSITIONING FOR FUNCTIONAL STABILITY

Upper and lower wax occlusal rims are made on autopolymerised resin bases. The mandibular base is made so that it smoothly covers the abutment replicas and attached healing caps. Holes in the plate and a recess in the rim may alternatively be provided (Fig 9-2). This clearance from contact with implants is necessary when the trial denture is tested for functional stability. Before mounting on the articulator, the sides of both casts are tapered to provide a denture remount facility (Fig 8-2).

Analysis of denture bearing foundations

The number and arrangement of artificial teeth used in overdentures should not be a preconceived preference. Mouths should be individually assessed for their ability to support prostheses.

The situation where a lower complete denture has poor foundations in the form of a resorbed jaw, while the maxillary denture is more adequately supported is a common one. In such mouths it is usually the lower prosthesis which will be implant retained. The design strategy is one which favours the prosthesis which is supported by the poorest foundation. As far as is possible occlusal forces generated between dentures are directed to consolidate the position of what is potentially the least stable denture, which in this case is the mandibular one.

THE CONSTRUCTION OF IMPLANT SUPPORTED LOWER AND CONVENTIONAL COMPLETE UPPER PROSTHESES

Usual crest of the ridge lines are augmented by left and right mandibular ridge profile lines drawn on the sides of the cast. A pair of modified compasses is useful but not essential for this (Fig 9-3 a). The lowest and flattest area of each profile line is identified and the extent of this marked with bisecting lines (Fig 9-3 b).

Denture stability is increased when the occlusal surfaces of teeth follow the surface contour of the underlying bone. The process is one of arranging the occlusal plane to follow the surface contour of the residual ridge beneath. This simple

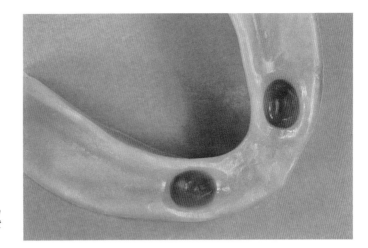

Fig 9-2 *Lower plate and wax rim with clearance from abutment replicas and healing caps.*

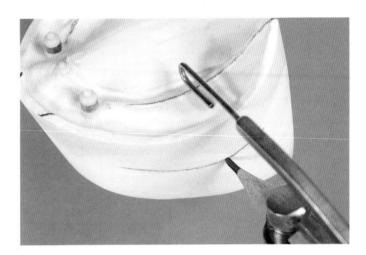

Fig 9-3 a *Modified compasses drawing a line which follows the profile of the residual ridge.*

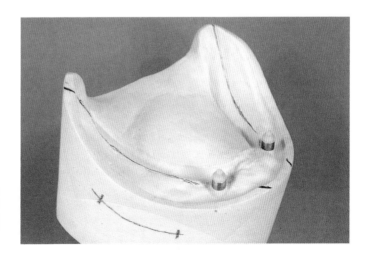

Fig 9-3 b *The ridge profile line bisected to show the flattest and most stable ridge part. Note the typical overall forward slope of the residual ridges.*

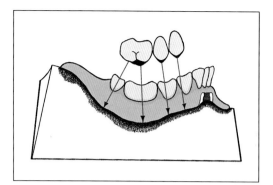

Fig 9-4 a   *The occlusal surfaces of posterior teeth should follow the shape of the dentures underlying bone foundation.*

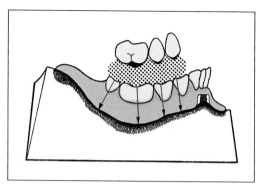

Fig 9-4 b   *The stable denture transmits occlusal forces at right angles to its supporting bone.*

mechanical rule ensures that occlusal forces arriving at right angles to the occlusal surfaces of the teeth are applied perpendicular to the bone; an arrangement which promotes stability in the tooth apart – denture under load situation (Figs 9-4 a and b).[2,3,4]

TOOTH MATERIALS

Acrylic resin materials are preferred because of their shock absorbing properties and ease by which teeth are provided with screw access holes. Since overdentures do not have screw holes and rest on mucosa, teeth may be resin or porcelain as clinically necessary. This license may not apply to teeth closely adjacent to implant and retainer parts. Depending on the size and position of these, a good deal of tooth reduction accommodation grinding may be necessary which precludes the use of porcelain.

SETTING–UP THE TEETH

After the upper anterior teeth have been set, the lower left and right first molar teeth are then positioned over the identified 'lowest' and, therefore, most 'stable' area of their respective ridge parts (9-Fig 5 a). Occlusal loads applied to teeth in this area will not act to displace the denture, regardless of residual ridge deficiencies. The situation is interestingly analogous to the way a saddle is positioned on a horses back. Saddles or teeth set elsewhere would not be as stable (Fig 9-5 b).

The remaining lower posterior teeth are then placed with regard to the fixed position of the first molar teeth. As well as a bucco–lingual centring over the ridge crest, their occlusal surfaces are arranged to follow the curve of the marked ridge profile lines (Fig 9-6 a). If, as is often the case in resorbed jaws, the ridge rises more steeply as it approaches the retro–molar pad, teeth set here would rest on a greater incline. Although loads applied perpendicular to occlusal surfaces would not cause denture movement, different

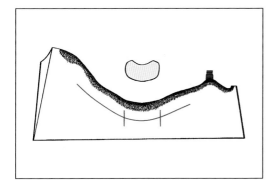

Fig 9-5 a *The first molar tooth is placed over the identified lowest and, therefore, most stable part of the ridge.*

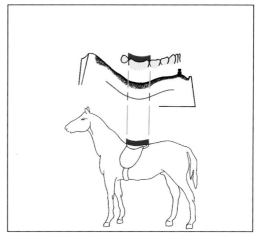

Fig 9-5 b *The analogy of a saddle on a horses back and a tooth over the lowest part of a resorbed ridge. Positions designed to achieve stability under dynamic load. After Gerber A. Complete dentures (IV).*[2]

occlusal pressures in this region would more easily displace the prosthesis where elsewhere more stable tooth positions exist (Fig 9-1).

This potential for instability is removed by omitting the second molar tooth or, alternatively, replacing it with a premolar. This tooth only makes full contact with the last upper tooth in protrusion. An occlusal contact which acts to stabilize the lower prosthesis, providing that the upper denture is satisfactorily secure (Fig 9-6 b).

If the upper prosthesis is not so endowed then these teeth are omitted too. It is always better to omit a tooth if its presence contributes to denture instability. Complete dentures resting on resorbed residual ridges are always more stable when the posterior teeth are confined to more horizontal ridge parts.

After the upper and lower posterior teeth have been set, lower incisor and canine teeth are selected and set to occupy the gap formed between the left and right lower first premolar teeth.

At the try—in of the dentures the dentist tests for functional stability without connection to the implants. Using a firm pressure from a pointed instrument, the occlusal surfaces of each posterior tooth is loaded, one side at a time. Regardless of which tooth is loaded the denture should not move during this test. When this stability has been confirmed, the position of the teeth adjacent to the implants is recorded by means of an imprint made in Lab—Putty (a). The trial prosthesis is now ready to receive its retention system to connect it to the implants.

OVERDENTURE RETENTION SYSTEMS

As well as those from implant manufacturers, there are independent suppliers of overdenture retention systems for use with most popular implants. These should be used with caution unless independent evidence of efficacy is also available.

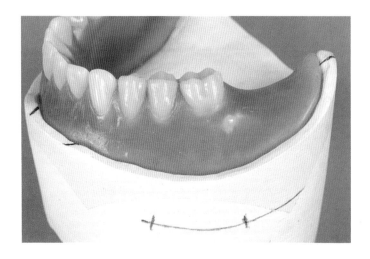

Fig 9-6 a *The occlusal surfaces of the teeth are arranged to follow the curve of the underlying residual ridge.*

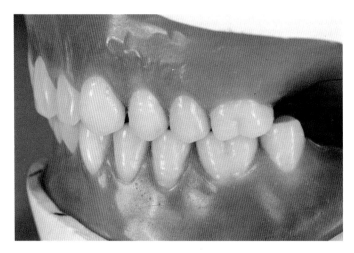

Fig 9-6 b *An extra premolar tooth may be used to stabilize the lower prosthesis during protrusive tooth contacts.*

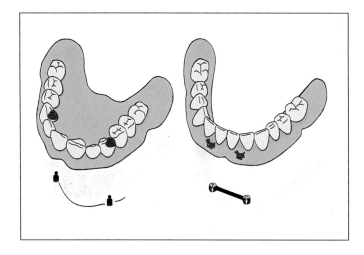

Fig 9-7 *Type 1 retainer (right). Prosthesis retained by clip connection to a bar joining two or more implants. Type 2 retainer (left). Prosthesis retained by connection to individual implants.*

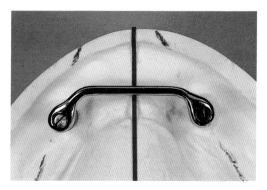

Fig 9-8 *Wrought bar with angled parts to bring the main straight onto the crest of the residual ridge and at right angles to the median axis (red line).*

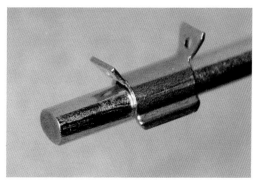

Fig 9-9 *Wrought overdenture gold bar and fitting retentive rider [clip].*

Also relevant is that implant manufacturers who have received recognition for implant use in one clinical situation may care to extrapolate this success to other products and applications, including overdenture retention systems.

Retention systems may be classified into two groups (Fig 9-7):

Type 1 Those where retainers contained in a prosthesis grasp a bar connecting two or more implants.

Type 2 Those where retainers contained in a prosthesis make connection with individual implants.

TYPE 1 RETAINERS

These bars are of lighter construction than the frameworks used for fixed prostheses. They are of a regular machined cross–section and span between implants, cantilevers are not usually provided. Overdenture bars should be positioned to occupy a straight line or as near a straight line as possible between implants and at right angles to the median axis. When a completely straight bar is not possible, the bar is bent with a main straight made parallel to the frontal occlusal plane, and subsidiary angled parts (Fig 9-8). Curved bars may be less satisfactory. Under functional denture movements, curved bars act to distort and possibly damage clips remotely positioned, relative to the median line (Chapter 12).

Articulated Retention Grip Bars (b)

These consist of a 1.90 mm diameter round wrought gold bar and riders [retention clips]. The riders have internal surfaces which make a closely fitting spring clip connection to the bar (Fig 9-9). Having selected a bar of the nearest suitable length (Chapter 14), this is shortened as necessary before bending to span the gap between the gold cylinders. A careful pliering is needed if nicks and other bar weakening blemishes are to be avoided. The bar is finally located either between the cylinders or on whatever cylinder side gives the best position relative to the

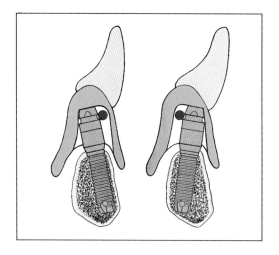

Fig 9-10 *Individual bar to gold cylinder positions may be altered to create increased space for the teeth and/or improved relationship to the underlying ridge.*

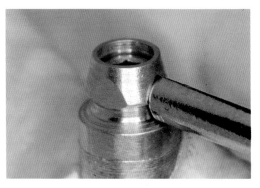

Fig 9-11 a *Bar in contact with a cylinder flat and resting on the lower edge of its circumferential groove.*

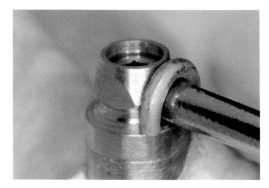

Fig 9-11 b *U shaped reinforcement wire fitting the bar and contacting the cylinder.*

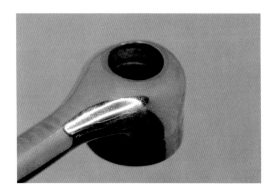

Fig 9-11 c *Completed wire reinforced soldered joint.*

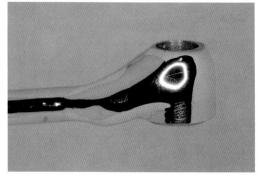

Fig 9-11 d *Soldered joint made on a cylinder provided with a cast type 4 gold alloy ledge.*

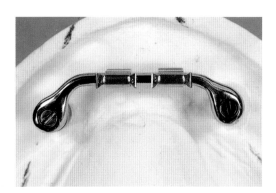

Fig 9-12 a *Finished wrought overdenture bar with attached clip retainers.*

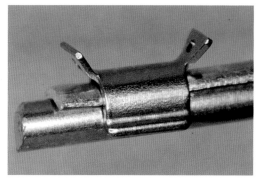

Fig 9-12 b *Clip fitted to the bar with interposed soft metal distance–piece or spacer.*

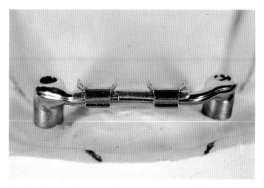

Fig 9-12 c *Clips in their correct position on the bar with spacer.*

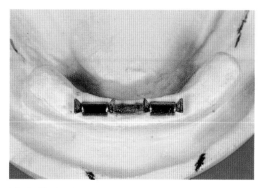

Fig 9-12 d *Clips, bar and spacer enclosed in plaster. Note protruding clip retention tags.*

ridge crest and teeth (Fig 9-10). Gold cylinders with different heights may be selected to equalize slight differences in abutment length. The final bar position is secured to cylinders using hard wax or Dura Lay resin, before investing in a soldering investment and joining the parts by solder (c). A joint of increased strength is obtained by placing 'U' shaped pieces of 1 mm gold wire on the bar in contact with the cylinders before soldering. This results in a substantially enlarged and consequently stronger joint (Figs 9-11 a–c).

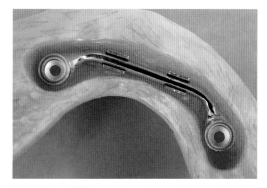

Fig 9-12 e *Fitting surface of overdenture showing clip to bar fitting.*

Alternatively, the cylinders may have small ledges cast upon them onto which the bar is then soldered. This can provide a very strong joint (Fig 9-11 d). The bar is supplied in an annealed state and requires heat treatment strengthening after soldering by holding it at a temperature of 400 °C for 15 minutes. A conventional porcelain furnace is ideally suitable for this work.

The resilient gold alloy riders, which clip onto the bar are supplied already strengthened so do not require further attention in this respect (Fig 9-12 a).

Most overdenture retention systems are supplied with a clip-to-bar spacer which is used during denture processing. When removed after polymerisation, the space formed allows a perpendicular denture movement/settling before complete rider to bar contact occurs (Fig 9-12 b). The soft metal spacer provided for this bar is 0.40 mm thick and is cut to length before placing between the clips and the bar (Fig 9-12 c). There is little agreement in the thickness of spacers supplied by different manufacturers and this variation should form part of their clinical selection (Chapter 14).

The bar, spacer and flexible sides of the clips are then encased in smoothed plaster, taking care not to cover the retention tags of the clips (Fig 9-12 d). The trial denture is then returned to its master cast and internally modified to sit over the plaster covering the retention system. Some tooth grinding alterations may be necessary in order to achieve this; work which precedes denture processing which then follows.

After grinding—in the occlusion (Chapter 8), the polymerised overdenture is removed from its master cast and the blocking—out plaster carefully picked out

with pointed instruments before polishing (Fig 9-12 e).

The clips are not adjusted for retention in the laboratory. Tools designed for the chairside tensioning adjustment and de—activation maintenance of riders are usefully available from the manufacturer.

Dolder bars

Many articles which appear in the literature propose the use of the Dolder bar retainer for complete overdentures, which is unfortunate. Dolder bars are unsuitable parallel sided rigid friction—grip devices. Dolder bar joints, by contrast, consist of an oval bar with resilient sleeve retainers, an arrangement which allows small tissue—wards denture movements, whilst maintaining retentive contact with the bar. The rigid connection of Dolder bars transmits all denture movement directly and without mitigation to the bar, its connectors, the soldered joints and implants (Fig 9-13 a).

Dolder bars must not be used in overdentures which are required to have limited movement under functional loads.

DOLDER BAR JOINT (b)

This wrought gold alloy bar is reduced in length as necessary to occupy as straight a line connection between the gold cylinders as is possible. The required configuration and cylinder to bar soldered joints duplicate that of the same manufacturers Articulated Retention Grip Bar, previously shown.

If closely adjacent joints are required, these may be made with S.G2 and S.G3 solders, the second of which has a 85 °C lower melting point than the first (b). Joint strength will again be substantially increased by U shaped wire reinforcement (Figs 9-11 a–c).

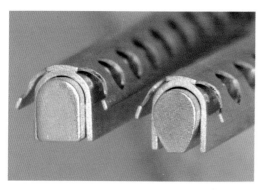

Fig 9-13 a *Left, parallel sided Dolder bar, right, Dolder bar joint.*

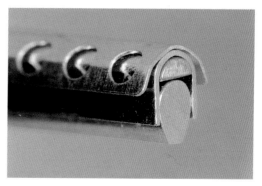

Fig 9-13 b *Spacer wire positioned between the Dolder bar joint and sleeve.*

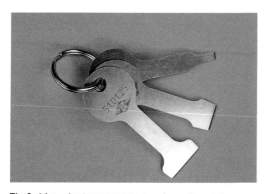

Fig 9-14 a *Instruments to tension clip retainers.*

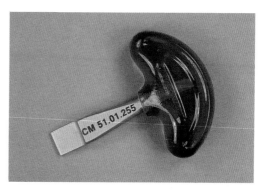

Fig 9-14 b *Tool to de–activate tensioned clips.*

After soldering and if S.G2 and S.G3 solders have been used, the bar is strengthened by heating it in a furnace at 400 °C for 15 minutes before polishing. If other solders are chosen the heat treatment requirements of the bar must be kept in mind.

The sleeve retainer is cut to length and a half–round spacer wire placed between an otherwise perfectly fitting sleeve and bar (Fig 9-13 b). The whole is then secured to place on the master cast using plaster. The under bar undercut is also blocked out with plaster, taking care that the sleeve

retention holes are not occluded. Two sizes of bar are available and the thickness of the provided spacer wire varies in accordance with the cross–sectional size of the bar selected (Chapter 14).

After processing and finishing the denture the sleeves are activated at the chairside by an inward bending adjustment of their sides, using tools made for the purpose. A sleeve de–activating device is also available (Figs 9-14 a and b).

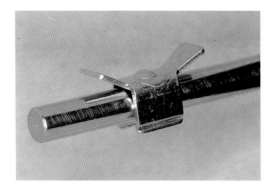

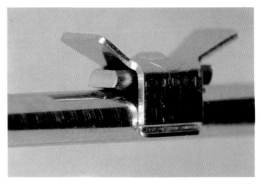

Fig 9-15 a (above left)   *Nobelpharma wrought gold bar and fitting clip.*

Fig 9-15 b (above right)   *Nobelpharma clip with positioned spacer wire.*

Fig 9-15 c   *Nobelpharma plastic pattern and attached clip.*

OVERDENTURE KIT WITH GOLD BAR (d)

These are available in two types, a wrought 2 mm diameter round gold alloy bar, 30 mm long, ready for use and a plastic pattern of the same dimensions for casting. Accompanying gold alloy retainer clips have spacer wires which allow 0.75 mm of denture movement/settling before a maximum clip to bar contact occurs. The same clips are used for both cast and wrought bars (Figs 9-15 a–c).

Cast bar

The plastic pattern is cut to length and joined to the gold cylinders with sufficient hard wax to make a strong joint. A sprue will be attached to each gold cylinder/bar junction. Always a concern is the remoteness of the centre bar parts from the sprues and the increased risk of contraction porosity arising from this. The pattern, complete with gold cylinders, is then invested and cast using the materials and methods described in Chapter 7, which includes strenghtening heat treatment. The finished assembly must satisfy the Sheffield one screw fitting test.

For some time the plastic pattern for these bars has inadvertently been provided with a diameter of 2.25 mm, a size which can damage the clips unless the bar has been reduced to the correct 2 mm diameter, either before or after casting. This reduction is very difficult if not impossible to achieve accurately. The first thing to be checked if clips used on cast

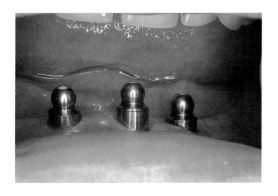

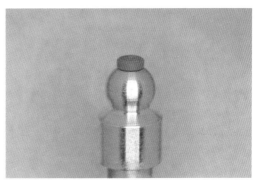

Fig 9-16 a *Nobelpharma ball attachments connected to standard titanium abutments.*

Fig 9-16 b (above right) *Abutment replica with removable plastic spacer.*

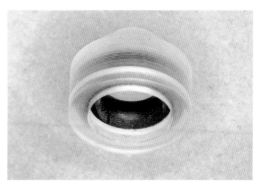

Fig 9-16 c *Plastic cup with contained resilient O ring.*

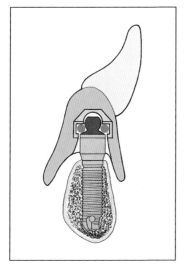

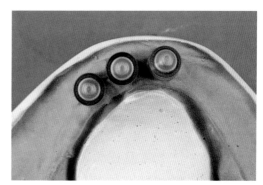

Fig 9-16 e *The cups can be too large to be used in some resorbed jaws.*

Fig 9-16 d *The connection of the O ring (green) with the ball attachment (red).*

bars become loose or fracture in service is that the cast bar is of the correct diameter (Chapter 12).

Wrought bar

These 2 mm diameter bars are used in the same way as the Articulated Retention Grip Bars made by the Cendres & Metaux Company. No post—soldering heat treatment bar strengthening is recommended by the Nobelpharma Company, however.

TYPE 2 RETAINERS

BALL ATTACHMENT (d)

The ball attachment consists of two parts, a titanium ball which is screw connected to standard abutments, an abutment replica with removable plastic processing spacer 0.60 mm thick, and a plastic cup with contained resilient O—ring. When correctly incorporated in the denture the cup and ball join to provide a resilient denture to implant connection (Figs 9-16 a–d).

Although the ball retainers are conveniently small, the cups have a diameter of 7.20 mm, a width which can be difficult to accommodate in some dentures (Fig 9-16 e). The O—rings need to be replaced periodically and this is usually done at the chairside.

INCORPORATING RETENTION SYSTEMS IN DENTURES

The enclosure of implants and retention systems within prostheses can weaken them to an extent where strengthening is necessary. Fortunately, a cast cobalt—chromium part lingual flange is easily incorporated in the denture, with the advantage of adequate strength in thin section.

Severe problems of overdenture bulk and tongue crowding occur when fixtures are malplaced or long abutment cylinders have been used. Altered bar positions, 3 mm gold cylinders and angulated abutments may help but the 5.5 mm height of the required conical gold cylinders somewhat less so.

After the retention system has been installed, the now complete trial denture is again tested in the mouth before processing.

PROCESSING AND FINISHING

Casts are removed from the articulator by tapping the exposed plaster/model junction with the handle of a plaster knife. An applied petroleum jelly lubrication of the exposed model sides before investing ensures their easy removal from the processing flask and their return to the articulator.

Grinding-in the occlusion

Acrylic resin contracts on polymerisation and this disturbs the obtained occlusion of the teeth. Because overdentures are most often used where the residual ridges are resorbed, overdentures tend to be large and resin contraction correspondingly greater. Resin films between the flask halves have a largely opposite effect in increasing the vertical dimension of the dentures.

These obstacles to occlusal balance are removed by tooth grinding with rotary instruments and the use of abrasive paste between the teeth as described in Chapter 8. The vertical incisal pin must contact the incisal guidance table when using grinding paste, especially with resin teeth. The alternative could be excessive tooth wear. The ground surfaces of porcelain teeth will require a final light rubber wheel polishing to restore their former lustre. The casts, articulator mountings and other records are then archived for possible future use.

REFERENCES

1. Jemt T, Book K, Linden B, Urde G. Failures and Complications in 92 Consecutively Inserted Overdentures Supported by Brånemark Implants in Severely Resorbed Edentulous Maxillae: A Study from Prosthetic Treatment to First Annual Check–up. *Int J Oral & Maxillofac Implants* 1992; 7: 162–167.

2. Gerber A. Complete Dentures (I). Quintessence International. Color Atlas. 1974; 7: 27–32.

   Ibid. Complete Dentures (II). The stability of maxillary dentures during mastication. 1974; 8: 27–32.

   Ibid. Complete Dentures (III). Better stability for mandibular dentures. 1974; 9: 31–36.

   Ibid. Complete Dentures (IV). The teamwork of dentures in chewing-function. 1974; 10: 41–46.

   Ibid. Complete Dentures (V). Functional dynamics determines the type of occlusion. 1974; 11: 43–47.

   Ibid. Complete Dentures (VI). Mastication- (ev. function-) centric for fit and tissue comfort. 1974; 12: 33–38.

3. White G E. The Gerber articulator and system of full denture construction. Part 1. The Condylator articulator. *Dental Technician* 1973; 26: 12–20.

   Part 2A. The impression technique and jaw registration. *Dental Technician* 1973; 26: 23–27.

   Part 2B. Setting-up the teeth and finishing the dentures. *Dental Technician* 1973; 26: 34–39.

4. Horn R, Stuck J. Zahnaufstellung in der Totalprothetik. 1980. Quintessence Verlags-GmbH. Berlin. (In German).

CHAPTER 9: MATERIALS AND EQUIPMENT

Manufacturer	UK Suppliers
(a) Lab-Putty	
Coltène AG	Coltène (UK) Ltd.
Feldwiesenstraße 20	8a Teknol House
CH-9450 Altstätten	Victoria Road
Switzerland	Burgess Hill
	RH15 9LF
(b) Articulated retention Grip Bar	
Dolder Bar Joint	
S.G2 and S.G3 solder	
Cendres & Metaux SA	Precious Metal Techniques
Route de Boujean 122	29 Chiltern Street
CH-2501 Biel-Bienne	London
Switzerland	W1M 1HG
(c) Deguvest L soldering investment	
Degussa AG	Degussa Limited
Postfach 110533	Winterton House
D-6000 Frankfurt 11	Winterton Way
Germany	Macclesfield
	SK11 0LP
(d) Overdenture Kit with Gold Bar	
Ball Attachment	
Nobelpharma AB	Nobelpharma UK Ltd.
Box 5190	Nobel House
S-402 26 Gothenburg	Packet Boat Lane
Sweden	Uxbridge
	UB8 2HG

Chapter Ten

The Construction of Maxillary Fixed Complete Prostheses

In mandibular treatment plans the position of fixtures is decided largely with prosthetic treatment in mind. In the maxilla the situation may almost be reversed. Here bone quality and its location is paramount, especially in the resorbed jaw. Fixtures will be installed wherever suitable bone and the treatment plan will allow. The implant scattering and tilting which can easily arise from this strategy can cause difficult screw access hole and framework design problems. Angulated abutments are immediately thought of in these circumstances but despite these, conditions can still exist in difficult cases which severly tax the invention of both technician and prosthodontist.

PROSTHESES WITH RESIN TEETH

When implants are arranged on, or in the front of the mouth slightly ahead of the ridge crest, an easy opportunity exists to design frameworks which duplicate those used in the mandible (Fig 10-1 a). Without the innervation restrictions of the mandible sufficient posterior fixtures may have been installed in the rear of the mouth,

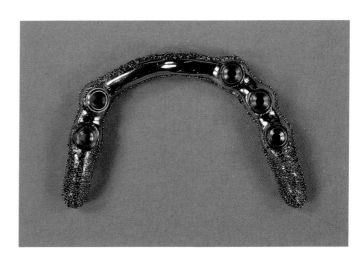

Fig 10-1 a   *Maxillary framework showing polished under—bar parts.*

169

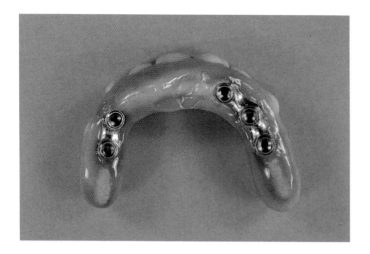

Fig 10-1 b *Prosthesis with resin extended to contact mucosal tissue anteriorly, with provided abutment cleaning space elsewhere.*

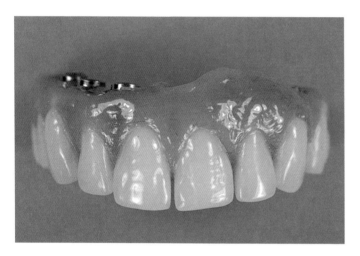

Fig 10-1 c *Appearance of labial flange.*

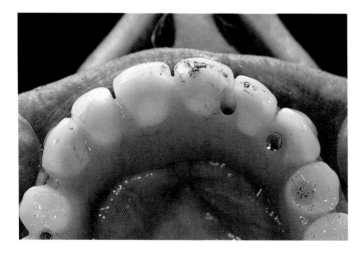

Fig 10-1 d *Soft tissue contact of resin before grinding to provide cleaning access space.*

which allow the framework to be entirely implant supported without cantilevering. This good fortune has the advantage of a wider and, therefore, potentially safer bearing. When distal cantilevering is necessary, this should be kept to a maximum length of 13 mm, whatever the bone quality or its maturity. When cantilevers are opposed by natural teeth, an implant supported prosthesis and/or 7 or 10 mm cantilever implants have been installed, cantilevers are restricted to a maximum length of 10 mm, with novice occlusal tables being shorter than this.

A space so carefully arranged beneath fixed mandibular prostheses for the purposes of cleaning access can be an embarrassment in maxillary dentures. Although the shortest abutments consistent with good oral hygiene access may have been used, unwelcome gaps between the prosthesis and soft tissues may still remain. If the patient has a high smile the space can be seen, and worse, patients may involuntarily 'whistle' or loose fluids through the gap.

Such difficulties are usually dealt with through the use of a developmental intermediate prostheses (Chapter 4). In final prostheses, such problems may be managed by allowing denture base resin to extend beneath the framework to closely approach the mucosa, whilst preserving a larger space around the abutments (Figs 10-1 b–d). As necessary, resin can be ground away to create more space as cleaning difficulties are encountered. Space enlargement using this method is gradual, with the patient more easily adapting to the increasing gap. If the framework is eventually exposed this will be of reduced importance if the framework has been previously polished (Fig 10-1 a).

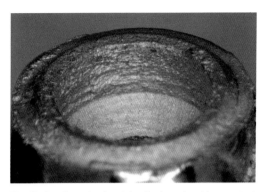

Fig 10-2 *Standard gold cylinder ruined by contact with molten metal–ceramic alloy.*

METAL–CERAMIC PROSTHESES

While it is true that resin teeth can have a good appearance and wear resistance, there is still a strong and increasing demand for porcelain bonded to metal prostheses, especially where prostheses occlude with natural teeth.

Although it is possible to make accurate metal–ceramic frameworks in one piece, the temperatures required for firing porcelain usually has the effect of distorting frameworks, especially larger ones. That many metal–ceramic alloys have melting ranges close to, if not exceeding those of standard gold cylinders and that superheating will increase these temperatures still further has already been discussed in Chapter 5. Cylinders may be damaged by contact with molten metal–ceramic alloy, sufficient to ruin their fitting surfaces (Fig 10-2).

SELECTION OF METAL– CERAMIC MATERIALS

Gold cylinders

Standard gold cylinders can be obtained in the same 1460–1500 °C melting range alloy used in the manufacture of the EsthetiCone cylinder (a). Alternatively, if the EsthetiCone abutment is used the accompanying cylinder allows metal–ceramic alloy/porcelain to be fused directly upon them, with a sub-gingival concealment of tooth margins (Chapter 11).

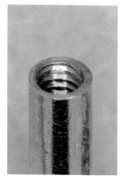 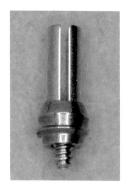

Fig 10-3 a (left)   Head Screw threaded tube.

Fig 10-3 b (right)   Screw with an elongated head and fitting collar.

Casting alloy and porcelain

There is no advantage in using metal–ceramic alloys for frameworks carrying resin teeth. When porcelain is fused on to a metal framework, an alloy with the highest safe liquidus temperature relative to the gold cylinders and the lowest fusing temperature porcelain is indicated.

Compound metal–ceramic constructions and one–piece type 4 gold alloy frameworks with added light cured resin teeth or cut down stock teeth are more easily and more accurately made. They also have the advantage of greater versatility and ease of maintenance.

THE CONSTRUCTION OF COMPOUND METAL–CERAMIC PROSTHESES

As an explanation of this method of construction an implant supported maxillary prosthesis opposed by lower natural teeth and tooth supported bridges will be considered.

Upper and lower master casts should be face–bow mounted on an articulator set to sagittal condylar path records.

Although average condylar path machines may be adequate for prostheses opposed by complete dentures, they may not be adequate when porcelain occlusal surfaces occlude with unyielding natural teeth or bridges.

Pattern making

Two sub–frame patterns incorporating standard gold cylinders are made using Dura Lay resin and hard inlay wax as described in Chapter 7. Also included are at least two Head Screw connectors per sub–frame (b). These connectors consist of a threaded tube and fitting collar which are connected by a screw possessing an elongated slotted head (Figs 10-3 a and b). The tubes are incorporated into the sub–frames with the intention of including them in the casting, together with the gold cylinders. Their correct position is where the screw will emerge within the occlusal surfaces of teeth, without forming occlusal stops for opposing cusps. Screw heads are eventually deformed and screwdriver slots closed by contact with natural teeth (Figs 10-8 b and c).

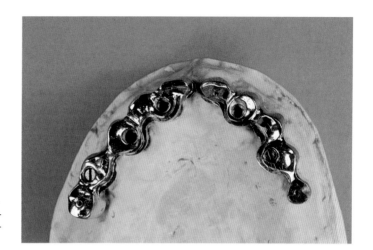

Fig 10-4 a *Cast Stabilor G sub—frames having machined surfaces developed in a parallelometer.*

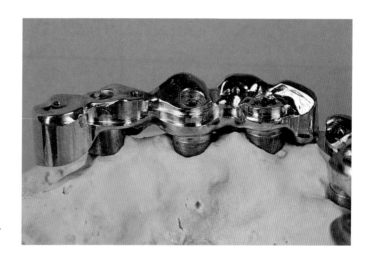

Fig 10-4 b *Detail of the patients right sub—frame showing vertical wall and horizontal ledge surfaces.*

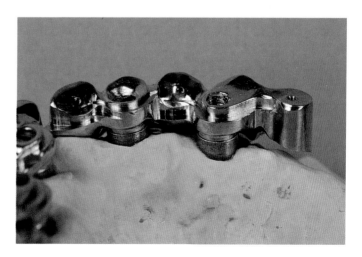

Fig 10-4 c *Detail of the left sub—frame.*

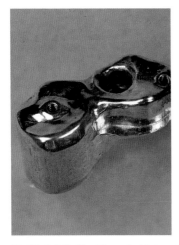
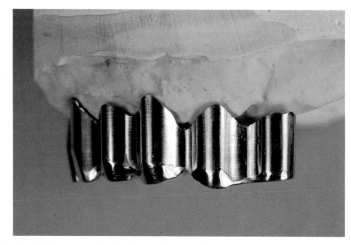

Fig 10-4 d (left) *Threaded tubes (Fig 10-3 a) incorporated in the sub—frame by casting—on.*

Fig 10-4 e (right) *Buccal surface of machine polished sub—frame with accurately parallel surfaces.*

Using a parallelometer the buccal and palatal surfaces of the sub—frames are shaped to have accurately perpendicular walls and horizontal ledges. The completed patterns must satisfy the Sheffield one screw fitting test before casting, using the materials and methods described in Chapter 7. Recovered castings are checked for a passive fit before returning to the parallelometer for final milling and polishing. A high degree of machining accuracy is necessary for this work (Figs 10-4 a–e).

The Head Screw collars are screw connected to the tubes in the sub—frames and Palavit GLC light cured resin (c) used to form removable shells approximately 0.5 mm thick (Fig 10-5 a). This material is

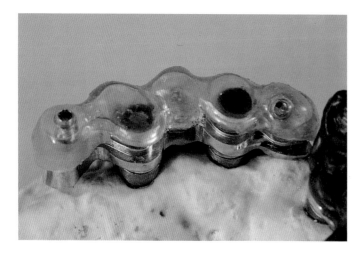

Fig10- 5 a *Light—cured resin shells made directly onto the sub—frames. Note included Head Screw collars.*

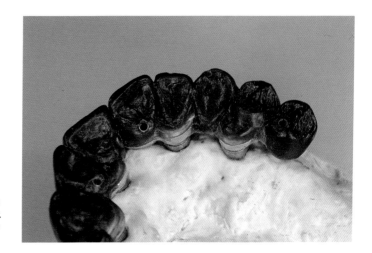

Fig 10-5 b *The final form of the teeth produced in hard inlay wax. Note the positions of the collars and threaded tubes.*

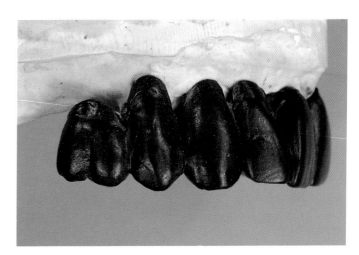

Fig 10-5 c *Finally developed shape and size of the teeth.*

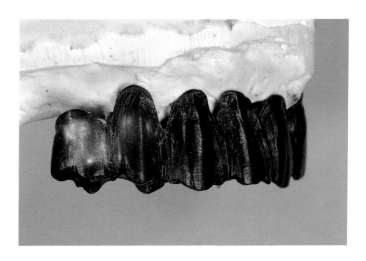

Fig 10-5 d *Wax pattern cut back sufficiently for the future casting to receive the correct thickness of porcelain.*

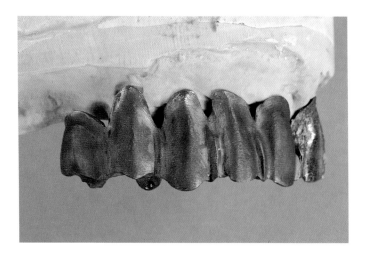

Fig 10-6 a   *Patterns cast in metal—ceramic alloy and fitted to the sub—frames.*

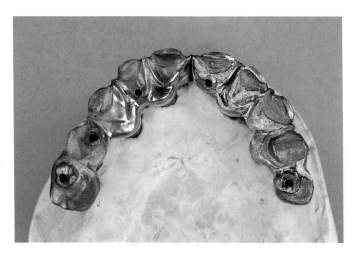

Fig 10-6 b   *Assembled castings showing future positions of connecting Head Screws.*

accurately stable when used in thin sections.

With the models in the articulator, inlay wax is added to the resin shells until the final shape of the anterior and posterior teeth has been achieved (Figs 10-5 b and c).

The final form of this work is recorded by imprinting in a bed of Lab—Putty (d) arranged on the lower frame of the articulator. By reference to this imprint, sufficient wax is then removed to allow an ade-

quate veneer thickness of porcelain (Fig 10-5 d).

Investing, casting and finishing

Using phosphate—bonded investment moulds the patterns are cast in metal—ceramic alloy. In the illustrated castings Ceramigold investment (e), was used with flame melted Matticraft E metal—ceramic alloy (f) cast into a mould leaving the furnace at 850 °C.

After checking their as—cast fit to the

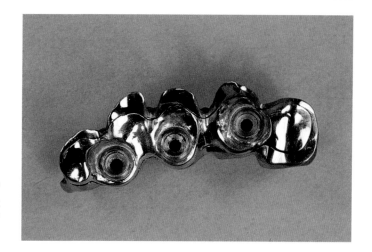

Fig 10-6 c *Metal–ceramic shell polished and fitted to its sub–frame without connecting screws. Note required close fitting of the parts.*

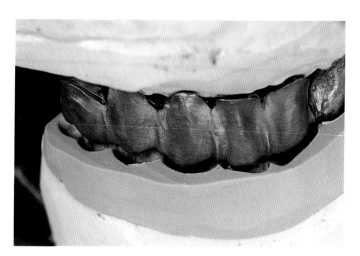

Fig 10-6 d *Lab Putty imprint of the waxed–up teeth which is used as a guide for the addition of porcelain.*

sub–frames the castings are prepared to receive porcelain which is added using the Lab–Putty imprint as a guide (Figs 10-6 a–d). Following porcelain firing, the completed work may then not completely fit the sub–frames. Engineers blue or other disclosing medium is then used for the identification and removal of what should be only small misfitting discrepancies (Figs 10-7 a and b).

After polishing, the finished metal–ceramic parts are connected to the sub–frames by the Head Screws (Fig 10-8 a). The screw heads are then reduced by grinding and polishing, to be inconspicuously flush with a provided small island of surrounding metal (Figs 10-8 b and c).

The final position of tooth necks relative to the mucosa is always a matter of compromise. Patients are usually pleased when this space is as small as possible, as this gives the best appearance. The cleaning access provided is less satisfactory (Fig 10-8 d).

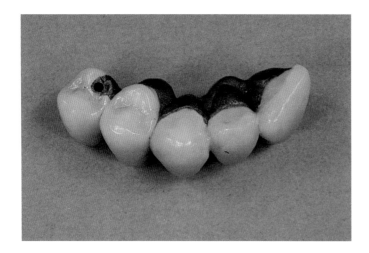

Fig 10-7 a *Appearance of metal–ceramic shell after addition of porcelain.*

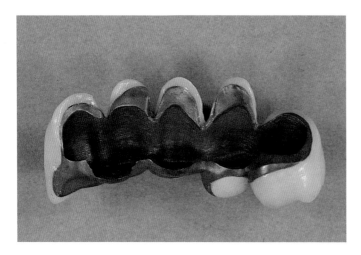

Fig 10-7 b *Ground fitting surface to correct porcelain firing induced misfitting.*

Fitting the prosthesis

Despite careful corrective grinding and complete absence of rocking or other fitting discrepancy, the metal–ceramic shell to sub–frame fitting may present a small gap at their margins. Provided that this space is small, this is of little importance as the shells fit the sub–frames and these in turn accurately fit the implants. If necessary, a closure gasket may be made at the chairside using silicone impression mate-

rial which is placed between the parts immediately before they are screw connected.

The sub–frames are installed in the mouth using standard gold screws. The metal–ceramic shells are then connected to the sub–frames using the already reduced Head Screws. Through the convenience of a compound construction and Head Screw connection, individual parts of the prosthesis are easily removable for alteration or maintenance, with teeth not

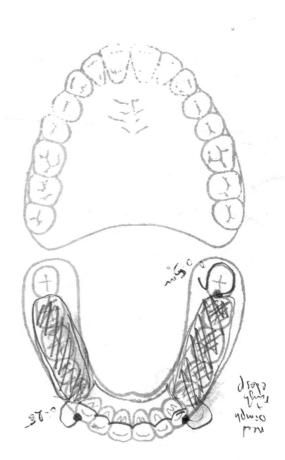

Mr. Fawcett

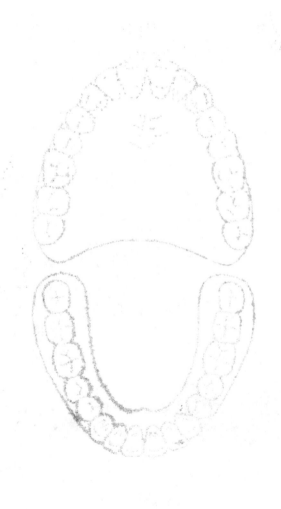

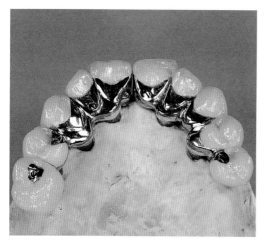

Fig 10-8 a *Finished compound prosthesis comprising four castings.*

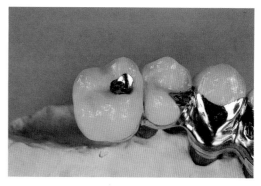

Fig 10-8 b *Screw heads reduced to be flush with island of surrounding metal contained in the occlusal surface of a porcelain tooth.*

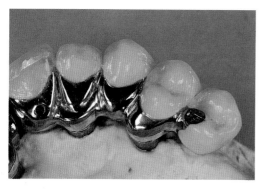

Fig 10-8 c *Palatal aspect of the prosthesis showing the disposition of porcelain, cast metal and implants.*

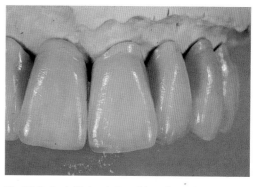

Fig 10-8 d *Initial relationship of tooth necks to mucosa. Following prosthesis insertion abutment cleaning access was then gradually enlarged until good oral hygiene was possible. The compound method of construction makes this process conveniently easy.*

spoiled by conventional gold screw access holes. The individual castings are of smaller size than would be required by a one—piece framework, so accuracy is improved, especially with the metal—ceramic parts.

PROSTHESES WITH ANTERIOR CANTILEVERS

In resorbed jaws a necessary forward setting of anterior teeth coupled with a bone finding rearward placement of fixtures may combine to require frameworks to then have anterior cantilevering (Figs

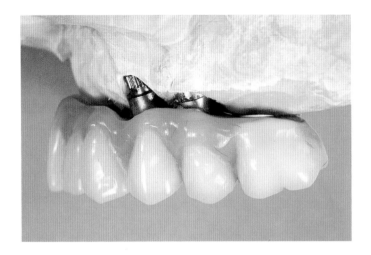

Fig 10-9 a *Prosthesis with anterior cantilevering of framework to allow the correct placement of incisor teeth.*

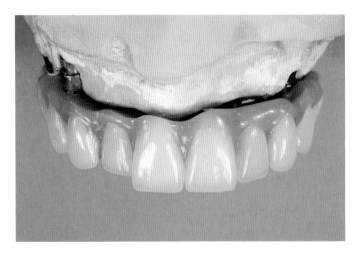

Fig 10-9 b *Appearance of prosthesis to mucosal tissue space. Compare with Fig 10-1 c and 10-1 d.*

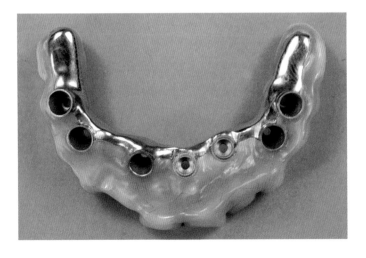

Fig 10-9 c *The resulting prosthesis has a substantial anterior cantilever and two distal extension cantilevers.*

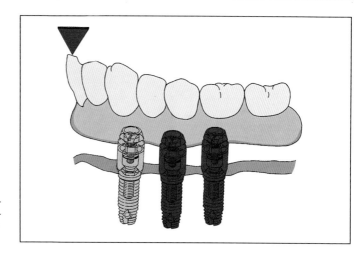

Fig 10-9 d *Loaded anterior cantilever showing implant compression (blue) and implant tension (red).*

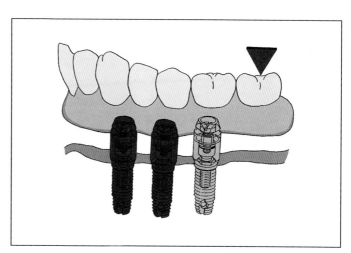

Fig 10-9 e *Loaded distal extension cantilever showing implant in compression (blue) and tension (red).*

10-9 a–c). A matter for concern is the long–term effect on implants and bone when anteriorly projecting cantilevers are combined with distal extension cantilevers. Through this addition the number of cantilever implants is now doubled, with each subjected to alternate compressive and tensile forces depending on which cantilever is bitten on (Figs 10-9 d and e). The long–term effect on bone and implant parts of such stress reversals is not known.

Frameworks with anterior cantilevers usually have an elongated shape, which is more difficult to cast accurately and dimensions which vary a good deal from one casting to another. Fortunately, their width and usually curved form combine to make an inherently strong shape. While some gold screws will have their access holes contained in teeth, others will be in exposed framework parts. Depending on framework thickness, screw heads may be either recessed in their metal access

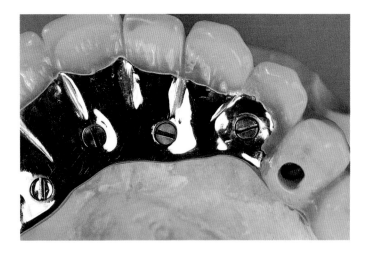

Fig 10-9 f   *Gold screws arriving flush with the surface of the framework are left polished.*

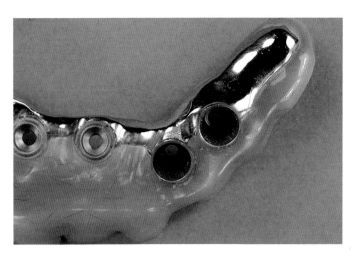

Fig 10-9 g   *Abutment access cleaning difficulties are increased when the prosthesis is widened by anterior cantilevering. Note the use of both standard and conical gold cylinders.*

holes and covered with composite filling material, or made flush with the surface and polished (Fig 10-9 f).

A recurring dilemma is the amount of abutment and under denture cleaning access space which should or can be provided as framework width increases (Figs 10-9 a, c and g).

The illustrated prosthesis was designed with a combination of Water Jet cleaning (g) and brush cleaning methods in mind.

CHAPTER 10: MATERIALS AND EQUIPMENT

Manufacturer	UK Suppliers
(a) Higher melting range standard gold cylinders	
Custom Manufacturing Division	Nobelpharma UK Ltd
Nobelpharma AB	Nobel House
Box 5211	Packet Boat Lane
S 402 26 Gothenburg	Uxbridge
Sweden	UB8 2GH
(b) Head Screw Connectors	
Cendres & Metaux SA	Precious Metal Techniques
Route de Boujean	29 Chiltern Street
CH-2501 Biel-Bienne	London
Switzerland	W1M 1HG
(c) Palavit GLC resin	
Kulzer & Co GmbH	Panadent Limited
Philipp-Reis-Straße 8	15 Great Dover Street
D-6393 Wehrheim /Ts	London
Germany	SE1 4YW
(d) Lab-Putty	
Coltène AG	Coltène (UK) Ltd.
Feldwiesenstraße 20	8a Teknol House
CH-9450 Altstätten	Victoria Road
Switzerland	Burgess Hill
	RH15 9LF
(e) Ceramigold investment	
Whip Mix Corporation	Skillbond Limited
361 Framlington Avenue	Dudley House
PO Box 17183	Gordon Road
Louisville	High Wycombe
Kentucky 40217	HP13 6EL
USA	

Manufacturer	UK Suppliers
(f) Matticraft E alloy Johnson Matthey Dental Materials Vittoria Street Birmingham B1 3NZ	
(g) Braun MD5 Water Jet Braun AG Frankfurter Straße 145 D-6242 Kronberg Germany	Braun (UK) Ltd Dolphin Estate Windmill Road Sunbury-on-Thames TW16 7 EJ

Chapter Eleven
The Partially Dentate Mouth

The success of implants in the edentulous mouth has led to intense activity to extend this to the partially dentate. When tooth loss is extensive, the required prosthesis may amount to a smaller version of that used in edentulous jaws. The situation changes when fewer teeth have been lost and/or these are in the front of the mouth. There may be less bone loss with the necks of natural and artificial teeth more easily apparent when smiling. Tooth and implant positions are now much more prescribed and the sight of abutments unacceptable.

The reasons why the partially dentate may seek implants are not necessarily the same as those who are edentulous. Problems of function and stability diminish as the number of replacement teeth becomes smaller. If treatment options include removable partial dentures, the lack of major connectors, clasps and soft tissue coverage may be sufficient reason for choosing implant support. When only a few teeth are missing and successful treatment by crowns or bridges could be expected, implants form but one of several reliable alternatives. A situation which does not apply to the edentulous patient.

Special care is necessary when implant supported prostheses are opposed by natural teeth. Implants are rigidly supported in bone and do not move under load. That which is tolerable by the implant and its bone bed may not be equally tolerable by opposing natural teeth. These may exhibit pain and sensitivity when in faulty contact with implant supported teeth. The closest attention must be given to the occlusion of the teeth especially when metal, metal–ceramic or ceramic tooth surfaces are to be provided. The use of an adjustable articulator is essential to undertake this work.

Despite the suitability of conventional bridges, the use of implant supported single crowns is increasing rapidly especially in younger patients. Primarily for maxillary incisors and canines and premolars in both jaws, they have the special advantage that natural tooth tissue is not destroyed or covered for the purposes of retention. The final crown and its implant 'root' have almost the same bulk as the natural tooth it replaces and its independence of adjacent teeth makes the creation of embrasures or diastemas simple.

Although standard abutments may be used anywhere in the mouth, anteriorly their appearance is usually unacceptable. In response to this need most implant manufacturers provide prosthetic components designed specially for single tooth restoration, consisting of a secure crown to implant fixation and concealed abutment.

New teams may easily assume that the single tooth restoration forms a convenient introduction to implant work. This is not the case. In edentulous jaws the correctly installed fixture has some latitude of required position, a tolerance which is virtually non–existent for implants in the front of the mouth. Appalling technical problems can occur when fixtures are malplaced with tooth position, length and emergence profile all severely compromised. A drilling stent will be required by even the most experienced surgeons (Chapter 3).

TREATMENT PLANNING

Using study casts, a wax–up of the proposed teeth or the use of altered resin stock teeth serves the dual purpose of indicating required fixture positions and showing the patient what is technically possible.

The height and width of the prosthetic components form an important patient selection criteria, especially when special abutments are used. If there is insufficient space for these parts implant support cannot be used. Study casts used in an adjustable articulator will confirm whether such parts can also be accommodated within excursive tooth contacts.

THE CERAONE ABUTMENT AND CROWN
(Nobelpharma AB, Sweden)

Only intended for single tooth replacement, the abutment has accurately parallel sides which makes it impossible to connect a single prosthesis to several CeraOne abutments. The crown to be replaced must have a neck width greater than 5 mm and a length greater than 5.25 mm to contain the abutment and prefabricated prosthetic parts. Smaller space than this and this abutment system cannot be used.

At what would usually be the abutment to fixture connection operation, a healing abutment is alternatively connected to the fixture. This has the same dimensions as the future abutment and crown neck, so essentially acts to 'pre–form' the healing gum to the correct final shape. Only after soft tissue healing does the patient return to have this replaced with a CeraOne abutment. Of octagonal cross–sectional shape, the abutment is available in 5 different collar heights the selection of which is related to mucosa thickness. By this clinical selection, crown margins may be placed sub–gingivally. A temporary restoration is then made to restore appearance and to maintain the mucosal form achieved (Figs 4-1 c and 4-8 c).

CeraOne alumina thimbles have an internal hexagon which fits the abutment and forms the foundation of an all–ceramic crown (Figs 11-1 a–d). Also with internally formed hexagons, plastic patterns are available for casting metal–ceramic crown copings (Fig 11-1 e).

The construction of ceramic CeraOne crowns

A special tray is made without an access window. The dentist then pushes a plastic impression coping onto the abutment in the mouth and cuts a hole in the tray so that its retaining tag then projects through (Fig 11-2 a).

Before the impression is removed from the mouth, the exposed tag is joined to the tray with autopolymerising resin

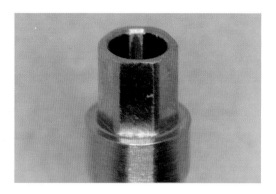

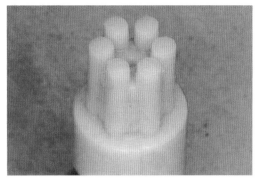

Fig 11-1 a *The clinical CeraOne single tooth titanium abutment.*

Fig 11-1 b *The plastic CeraOne abutment replica.*

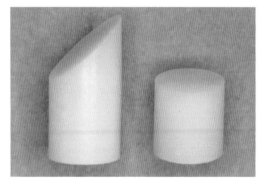

Fig 11-1 c *Alumina CeraOne thimbles are available in two external shapes, both having an internal hexagon which fits over the abutment.*

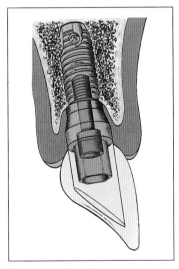

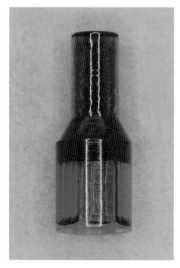

Fig 11-1 d *CeraOne crown system showing arrangement of abutment, ceramic thimble (green) and gold alloy abutment screw.*

Fig 11-1 e *Plastic pattern for casting metal—ceramic crown copings.*

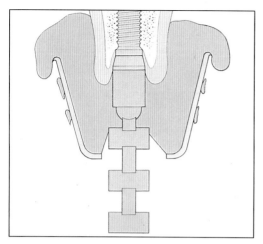

Fig 11-2 a *Impression of the CeraOne abutment in the mouth with tag of plastic impression coping protruding through the tray.*

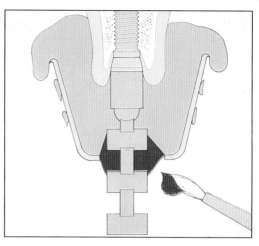

Fig 11-2 b *Coping joined to the tray with Dura Lay resin.*

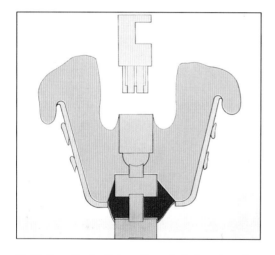

Fig 11-2 c *Push–fit insertion of abutment replica into the impression coping.*

Fig 11-2 b). The removed impression is immediately checked for a securely located coping. These have a tight fit in the mouth and a single path of withdrawal, so their attachment to the tray can be broken to cause an inaccuracy. A plastic abutment

replica is then inserted into the waiting coping. Care is needed here; this is also a push fit (Fig 11-2 c).

A necessary close contact between the neck of the crown and the mucosa is made easier when the model contains a soft mucosa replica made from Gi–Mask material (a).

The most appropriately shaped alumina thimble is tried on the abutment replica and its position with adjacent and opposing teeth checked. If necessary, its outer parts can be ground away with diamond instruments, but their final wall thickness must not be less than 0.50 mm. Although thimbles have a smooth outer surface it is not necessary to roughen this for porcelain retention; but they must be scrupulously clean before use.

It is careful practice, especially when implant positions are difficult, to try a wax crown of the proposed restoration in the mouth. When this is satisfactory, a Lab–Putty (a) mould is made, which then acts as a guide to the final crown.

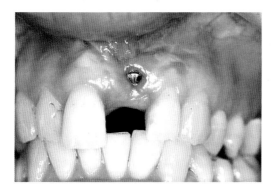

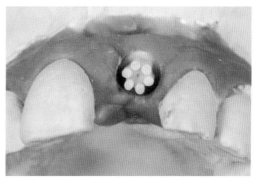

Fig 11-3 a *Exposed malplaced single tooth fixture before abutment connection.*

Fig 11-3 b *Stone cast with soft mucosa replica and plastic abutment replica.*

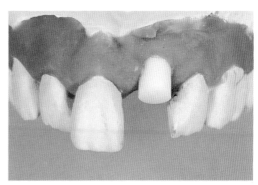

Fig 11-3 c *Positioned ceramic thimble showing inconvenient position for crown construction.*

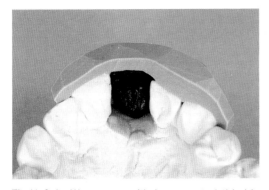

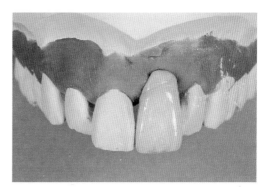

Fig 11-3 d *Wax crown with incorporated thimble contained in a two part Lab–Putty impression mould (palatal part removed).*

Fig 11-3 e *Finished porcelain crown with elongated neck.*

Core material, which should contain 45 %–50 % alumina, is then applied in two firings, the second 10 °C lower than the first. Other porcelains are added as necessary and fired as recommended by their manufacturer. No departure from usual crown and bridge porcelain work is required. The illustrated crown shows the difficulty of making a satisfactory tooth on an incorrectly placed fixture (Figs 11-3 a–e).

Knowing the technical difficulties

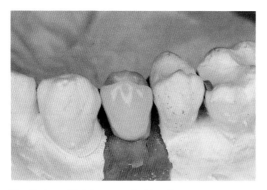

Fig 11-4 a *Metal–ceramic CeraOne crown.*

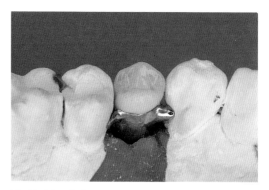

Fig 11-4 b *Palatal aspect showing optional metal extension wings contacting adjacent teeth.*

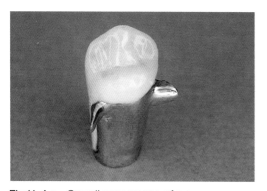

Fig 11-4 c *Overall appearance of crown.*

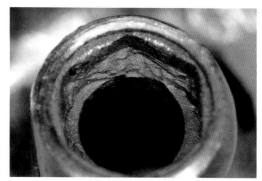

Fig 11-5 *An inaccurately cast hexagon made from an accurate plastic pattern.*

caused by misaligned fixtures, Nobel-pharma suggest that a space provided between the ceramic thimble and Cera-One abutment for the cement lute can be used to re–position crowns.[1] Even when forcibly tilted the displacement gap produced between the crown and the abutment is less than 0.08 mm wide, so is of little use in this respect. The angulated abutment cannot be used either, because a crown made on its tapered gold cylinder lacks rotational resistance.

Metal–ceramic CeraOne crowns

CeraOne plastic patterns are re–shaped as necessary, including the addition of wax before casting in metal–ceramic alloy. Porcelain is then added, following usual practice. Some workers choose to incorporate wing extensions on longer metal–ceramic crowns to provide extra stability (Figs 11-4 a–c). Whereas thimbles have finished fitting surfaces, patterns have internal hexagons which have to be

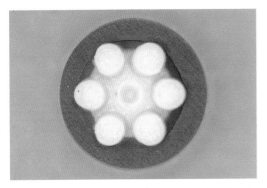

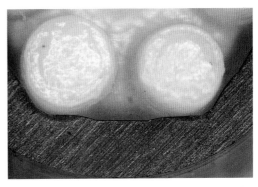

Fig 11-6 a *Sectioned plastic pattern placed onto the abutment replica showing its small area of fitting contact.*

Fig 11-6 b *Detail showing pattern to replica spaces.*

cast. If the angles forming these are only slightly less than accurate, the crown cannot be placed on the abutment in the mouth.

It has been shown that casting investments are not always able to adequately form angles contained in patterns and that pattern chamber walls can be damaged during metal entry to cause an even greater misfit. Phosphate—bonded materials, which must be used for metal—ceramic alloys, are particularly poor in this respect.[2] Investment mould inaccuracies are a source of misfitting wherever patterns containing internal angles have to be cast, including those of the UCLA plastic abutment type (Fig 11-5).[3] Manufacturers claim a high degree of fitting accuracy for their plastic patterns. Although this may well be the case, it overlooks the fact that the final fitting quality is decided by the technician who casts it. Knowing this, some manufacturers provide what are claimed to be fit—correcting grinding tools. Such devices have limited value, in that they are only able to cosmetically reduce rough metal at the marginal rim of

castings. They are not able to improve the fitting qualities of faulty internal hexagons.

The fit of metal—ceramic CeraOne crowns

Unfortunately, a crown of almost any quality will appear to have a satisfactory fit on the abutment replica. This is made of soft plastic and unlike its titanium counterpart comprises entirely rounded parts (Fig 11-1 b). Consequently, casting inaccuracies are easily accommodated within casting to replica spaces and replica compression, distortion or abrasion (Figs 11-6 a–c). With this fitting error concealment in mind, it is strongly recommended that a clinical titanium abutment be obtained for laboratory use. By using this the fitting quality of work can be accurately assessed at the bench before trial in the mouth (Fig 11-6 d).

In response to these difficulties Nobelpharma have now introduced part DCA 160 which is a cylinder or sleeve which accurately fits the plastic abutment and onto which metal—ceramic alloy can be

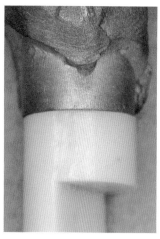

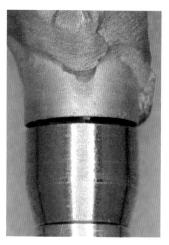

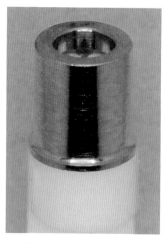

Fig 11-6 c *A metal–ceramic alloy casting with internal fitting surface defects having an apparent satisfactory fit on the replica.*

Fig 11-6 d *The casting fitting on a CeraOne titanium abutment showing an obviously poor fit.*

Fig 11-6 e *Gold sleeve which provides an accurate fitting surface for a cast metal–ceramic crown.*

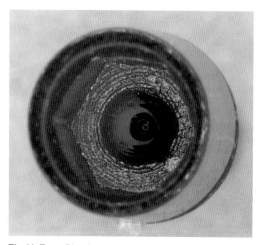

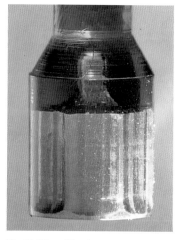

Fig 11-7 a *Plastic pattern showing an internal contraction pipe.*

Fig 11-7 b *Plastic pattern lit from inside showing size and shape of internal contraction pipe.*

cast. The gold alloy of its construction has a melting range of 1400 °C to 1490 °C and a machined bevel provides a metal–ceramic/porcelain finishing edge (Fig 11-6 e). Porcelain will not adequately adhere to the sleeve so a sufficient coverage of metal–ceramic alloy must be provided to obtain an adequate porcelain bond.

The CeraOne plastic pattern is sometimes affected by an internal contraction pipe on its fitting surface which should be

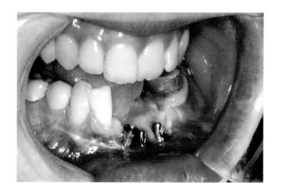

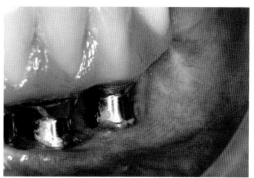

Fig 11-8 a above left) *Severe traumatic bone loss in the front of the mouth. Three fixtures two with angulated abutments installed.*

Fig 11-8 b (above right) *Resin teeth supported on a type 4 gold alloy framework. In these circumstances appearance is not compromised by an adequately wide under–denture cleaning space.*

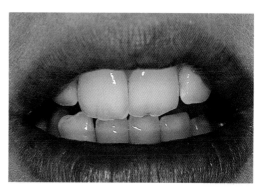

Fig 11-8 c *Youthful dental appearance which is not compromised even when the patient is smiling. It is not possible to see the abutments.*

avoided (Figs 11-7 a and b). When sharply pointed this produces an apex of investment in the mould, which can be abraded as metal flows over it. Investment fragments produced can be drawn into the metal causing contamination.

PARTIAL PROSTHESES

The materials and prosthetic components used in the edentulous mouth are also convenient for larger partial prostheses and for all restorations situated in the rear of the mouth. Where bone loss is sufficient that abutments will not be seen, standard abutments may be the preferred clinical choice. For example, where there has

been localised severe traumatic bone loss in an otherwise normal jaw, standard or angled abutments can be used in the front of the mouth, without compromising appearance and with good cleaning access (Figs 11-8 a–c). A continuing debate centres on whether implant supported prostheses should be connected to natural teeth or not. The weight of present opinion suggests that natural teeth should not be included, although this will be a clinical decision.

Partial prostheses may be conveniently classified by the materials used in their construction.
a) Prostheses where resin teeth are carried on a type 4 gold alloy framework.
b) Metal–ceramic prostheses.

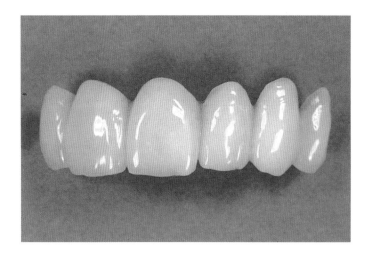

Fig 11-9 a *Appearance of anterior restoration with resin teeth.*

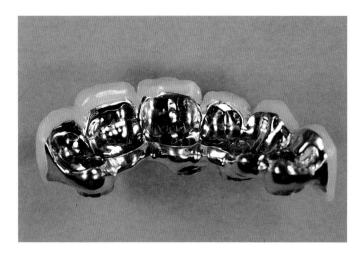

Fig 11-9 b *Framework made from type 4 gold alloy cast onto four standard gold cylinders.*

The construction of prostheses using type 4 gold alloy frameworks and resin stock teeth presents reduced difficulties of obtaining a passive fit. Porcelain stock teeth can also be used providing that it is not necessary to provide them with screw access holes, which is impossibly difficult.

As shown in Chapter 10, metal—ceramic castings tend to loose their fitting accuracy during the firing of porcelain. The larger the prosthesis and the greater the number of porcelain firings, the greater the misfitting caused. Tie bars joining distal framework parts will help reduce distortion but post—firing correction soldering is presently the only reliable method of dealing with this problem. Smaller prostheses are much more accurately made, however. Restorations carrying up to 4 or 5 teeth can be routinely made in one—piece, without soldering corrections.

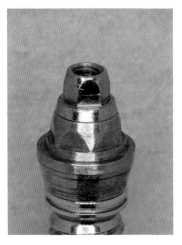

Fig 11-10 a *EsthetiCone abutment connected to a fixture.*

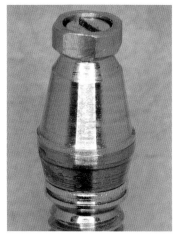

Fig 11-10 b *Conical gold cylinder screw connected to the abutment.*

PROSTHESES WITH RESIN TEETH

Either ground—down stock teeth or light—cured resin teeth may be used when constructing prostheses. As the framework does not need enlargement to support porcelain, those carrying resin teeth can be of smaller bulk, which saves alloy and improves casting accuracy.

Restorations in the front of the mouth will closely resemble metal—ceramic restorations, except that the fitting quality obtained will be more reliably accurate. Although the teeth will eventually need replacement, this work can be easily undertaken without framework revisions (Figs 11-9 a and b).

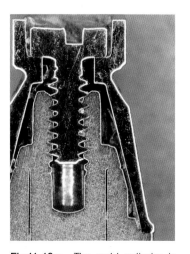

Fig 11-10 c *The gold cylinder is centred by its gold screw and contacts the abutment only at its rim.*

THE ESTHETICONE ABUTMENT (Nobelpharma AB. Sweden)

The EsthetiCone tapered abutment uses a conical and higher melting—range gold cylinder, onto which metal—ceramic alloy can be cast. An external marginal chamfer provides a usefully necessary framework/porcelain finishing edge (Figs 11-10 a–c). The abutment is screw connected to standard fixtures and is used for

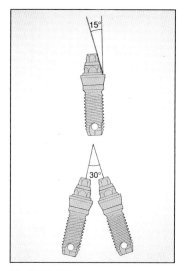

Fig 11-11 *The abutment and its abutment screw form a taper which allows implants forming angles of up to 30° to still allow prosthesis connection.*

restorations supported by two or more implants, up to and including complete prostheses. The abutment comprises a collar and abutment screw head, which together forms an overall taper of 15°, an angulation which allows tilted fixtures with included angles of up to 30° to allow prosthesis insertion (Fig 11-11).[4]

Fixture position

The minimum usable space between the fixture terminal and opposing teeth is 6.7 mm. If there is less space than this the EsthetiCone abutment cannot be used (Fig 11-12 a). For the best crown appearance the connecting terminal of the fixture must be related to the cemento—enamel junction of the adjacent teeth. When sub—gingival porcelain margin concealment is required, the height of the abutment and the positional height of the fixture terminal must be related to soft tissue thickness.

Fig 11-12 a *The EsthetiCone abutment cannot be used if there is less than 6.7 mm between the fixture and opposing teeth.*

Fig 11-12 b *The relationship between fixture position, mucosa thickness and the cemento—enamel junction of the teeth, decided at the time of fixture installation, controls the sub—gingival position of crown margins.*

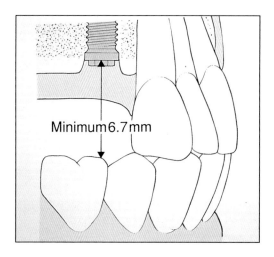

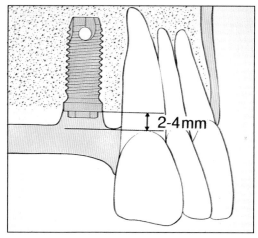

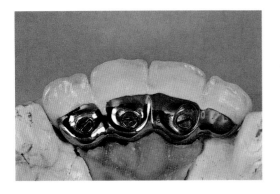

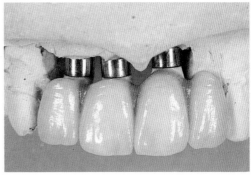

Fig 11-13 a (above left) *Completed metal—ceramic prosthesis with implants in helpful positions.*

Fig 11-13 b (above right *Abutment access and visibility are improved on removing the mucosal insert.*

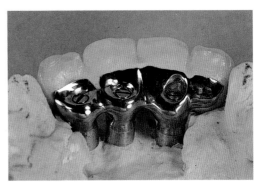

Fig 11-13 c *Palatal sub—gingival metalwork showing rounded form.*

The best appearance will be obtained only when fixture position, mucosa thickness, abutment collar height and gold cylinder height are accurately co—ordinated (Fig 11-12 b).

Apart from its connecting gold screw, the EsthetiCone gold cylinder has contact with its abutment only at its rim, so can rotate in use. For this reason it cannot be used for single teeth.

THE CONSTRUCTION OF METAL—CERAMIC PROSTHESES USING ESTHETICONE ABUTMENTS

The master cast may usefully have a Gi—Mask mucosa replica insert which is removable. This is advantageous in that the fit of more complex work can be more easily seen and tested and access for sub—gingival porcelain work improved (Figs 11-13 a—e). The illustrated prosthesis was made in one piece using Herabond E alloy (b), cast into a Ceramigold phosphate—bonded investment mould (c). The investment was mixed with 50% room temperature water and 50% manufacturer provided special liquid. Although this prosthesis was accurately made in one—piece using Duceram porcelain (b), Herabond pre—bonding and post—bonding corrective solders are also available (Chapter 14). This prosthesis was made for the mouth shown in Fig 3-3 c.

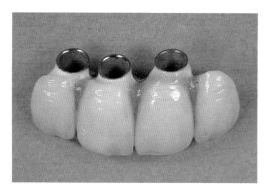

Fig 11-13 d   *Overall form of the finished prosthesis.*

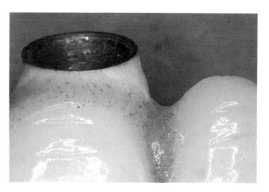

Fig 11-13 e   *Porcelain can be brought to the marginal rim of the cylinders, see Fig 11-10 b.*

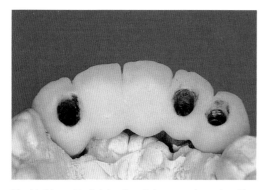

Fig 11-14 a   *Unfinished metal—ceramic restoration showing correctly placed screw access holes in porcelain.*

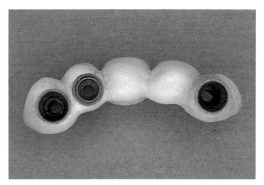

Fig 11-14 b   *Provisional form of the restoration showing complete enclosure of metalwork. Note accurately helpful placement of implants.*

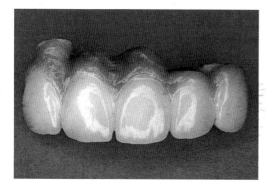

Fig 11-14 c   *Finished restoration with applied porcelain gum—work.*

The illustrated prosthesis demonstrates the need for accurate fixture placement if gold cylinders are to be correctly contained within individual tooth crowns, the prosthesis is to have the smallest bulk and best appearance be obtained (Figs 11-14 a–e). Pink porcelain reduces an otherwise necessarily elongated crown length, but providing this requires care. Abutment cleaning access can be easily compromised if this is overdone.

It can be seen that the central gold

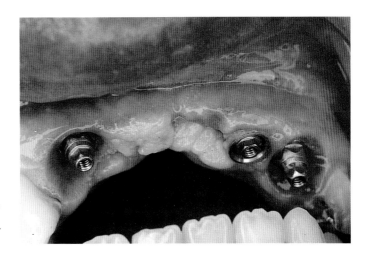

Fig 11-14 d *Mouth ready to receive the finished restoration. Note the pre—formed soft tissues around the EsthetiCone abutments.*

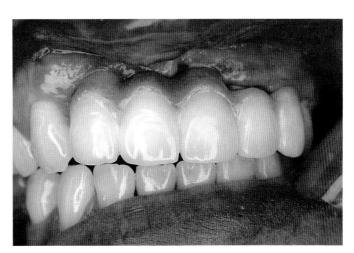

Fig 11-14 e *Installed prosthesis with accurately coloured gum—work.*

cylinder is a standard cylinder. Careful temperature control is necessary when casting metal—ceramic alloy onto standard cylinders, if severe damage is to be avoided (Fig 10-2).

An attractive proposition for the larger restoration is to provide a fixture for each missing tooth. Although the crowns would have to be connected by a framework, the procedure amounts to the placement of multiple single tooth implants in the same jaw. The consequences of imperfect fix-

ture positioning in such work ranges on a scale between difficulty and disaster. This treatment approach is entirely the domain of the most experienced and skilful implant teams.

THE FITTING OF PROSTHESES

CeraOne crowns are cemented in place in the mouth while prostheses supported by EsthetiCone abutments are secured by gold screws. Although providing easy retrievability, screw fixation carries the disadvantage that teeth can be marred by visible access holes. These problems are best dealt with at the chairside, using tooth filling materials.

Since there is a gap between the EsthetiCone abutment and its cylinder, gold screws have the important additional function of centring the bridge onto the abutments (Fig 11-10 c). Any fitting error in the construction in excess of approximately 0.08 mm will immediately be applied to the gold screws, implants and bone on tightening (Table 5-5). The likely damaging effect of such stresses have already been described in Chapter 5. The clinician has the added difficulty of assessing the fit of prostheses which have margins placed sub—gingivally. Only a radiographic assessment is possible in these circumstances and this is not as reliable and accurate as a visual examination.

REFERENCES

1. CeraOne Abutment — Esthetical Single Tooth Replacement. Technique booklet PRI 183 91.02. Nobelpharma AB, Gothenburg, Sweden.

2. White G E. The Resistance of Selected Dental Casting Investments to Casting Stresses. PhD Thesis, University of Sheffield. 1987.

3. Lewis S, Beumer J, Hornburg W, Moy P. The 'UCLA' Abutment. *Int J Oral & Maxillofac Implants* 1988; 3: 183–189.

4. EsthetiCone Abutment — Esthetical Restorations Procedure. Technique booklet PRI 182 91.06. Nobelpharma AB, Gothenburg, Sweden.

CHAPTER 11: MATERIALS AND EQUIPMENT

Manufacturer	UK Agents

(a) Gi–Mask
Lab–Putty
Coltène AG
Feldwiesenstraße 20
CH-9450 Altstätten
Switzerland

Coltène (UK) Ltd
8a Teknol House
Victoria Road
Burgess Hill
RH15 9LF

(b) Herabond E alloy
Duceram porcelain
Heraeus Kulzer GmbH
Postfach 1552
6450 Hanau
Germany

Chaperlin and Jacobs Limited
No. 1 Four Seasons Crescent
Kimpton Road
Sutton
SM3 9QR

(c) Ceramigold investment
Whip Mix Corporation
361 Framlington
PO Box 17183
Louisville
Kentucky 40217
USA

Skillbond Limited
Dudley House
Gordon Road
High Wycombe
HP 13 6EL

Chapter Twelve
Maintenance and Repairs

Because treatment objectives are long—term ones, virtually all prostheses will eventually require some remedial attention; this may depend on the materials used in their construction. Resin denture parts eventually wear away and experience has shown that this is more common when oral hygiene procedures are practiced vigorously.

Occasionally, prostheses require modification in order to provide easier cleaning access when the wearer has suffered a loss of manual dexterity or other impairment. New patients may also fail to clean their prostheses properly. This problem will need to be remedied by patient re—instruction or prosthesis modification, or both. In either event the prosthesis will be returned to the laboratory for cleaning. This is easily achieved using a stain/tartar removing solution in an ultrasonic cleaning bath. It becomes apparent that in some areas deposits occur more frequently. These are the areas where new prostheses need to be made as smooth and 'self cleansing' as possible (Figs 12-1a and b).

Patients who were pleased to have a dental appearance based on reduced cleaning access at tooth necks or abutment cylinders may find the same prosthesis less convenient in later years. Whether the prosthesis should or can be modified or, alternatively, should a new more suitable prosthesis be made for older and perhaps infirm patients, are difficult decisions which will have to be increasingly addressed in the future.

The ease by which prostheses can be dealt with depends in the first instance on the keeping of a archive. If prescription cards, models and articulator mountings have been stored and indexed, then this work is greatly facilitated. Also useful with regards indexing is the automatic imprinting by some articulators of their serial numbers onto work (Fig 8-1b). Difficulties arise when patients present work undertaken elsewhere and such information is not available.

The bone height around implants is checked annually. If yearly losses much in excess of 0.1 mm are discovered, this will be taken as an urgent signal that a fault exists in the design or construction of the prosthesis.[1] The prosthesis will be removed and checked for a passive fit in the mouth. Archived master casts may not be particularly helpful if they contain inaccurate or damaged replicas (Chapter 5).

When implant parts fracture or become loose or prosthetic components fail, a full explanation for this occurrence should be obtained before any repair is contemplated. It is not sufficient to restore that which should not have failed.

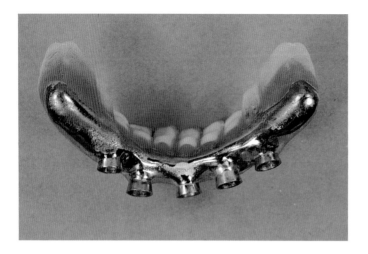

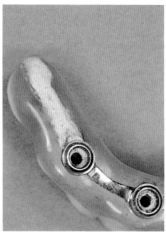

Fig 12-1 a (above left) *New prosthesis with tartar deposits on lingual and under parts due to poor oral hygiene.*

Fig 12-1 b (above right) *Tartar deposit under a cantilever made with inadequate cleaning space.*

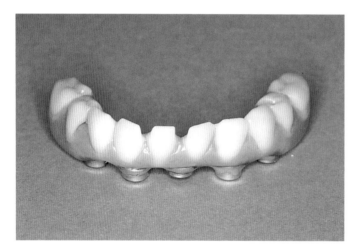

Fig 12-1 c *Worn denture showing overall loss of tooth and denture base material.*

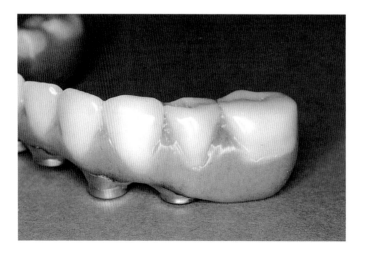

Fig 12-1 d *If the patient is right—handed the right side of the denture often shows increased wear.*

THE REPLACEMENT OF WORN ACRYLIC TEETH AND DENTURE BASE

This is a usual and expected travail. Worn dentures are characterised by a loss of surface detail, affecting both teeth and denture base (Figs 12-1 c and d).

When the original master cast is available this is returned to the articulator, together with a model of the opposing dentition. An opposing complete denture will be remounted, in preference to a cast of this prosthesis. Usually, the original vertical dimension will not have been lost and this can be confirmed by reference to the height scale of the articulators incisal guidance pin.

When a master cast is not available, used replicas are screw connected to the framework and these embedded in stone to make a repair model. The prosthesis is then occluded directly with the opposing teeth or via a jaw registration wafer record taken before mounting on the articulator. Using tweezers the removed worn prosthesis is held over rather than placed in a Bunsen flame. After a few moments heating and possibly burning, the hot resin can be peeled off using a second pair of tweezers. The framework and contained gold cylinders will not be damaged by this heat. The revealed framework is then ultrasonically cleaned in a stain remover solution, followed by a light mechanical polishing to restore its original lustre.

The setting of replacement teeth and re—waxing precedes trial in the mouth. The denture is finished in heat cured resin and lightly ground—in to the opposing model or denture using the original articulator settings.

FRACTURE OF DENTURE BASE RESIN

Any repair confined to the resin base must be thought of as temporary, in that the fracture will almost certainly re—occur. In fixed prostheses the underlying cause of the problem can usually be traced to a faulty framework. When the problem occurs adjacent to cantilevers, it is almost certainly related to an inadequate strength and/or length of these highly stressed framework parts (Figs 12-2 a and b). If the framework is too thin overall it will have to be re—made. If the casting is otherwise satisfactory but the cantilever is either too short or too thin, then the cantilever repair described later in this chapter may suffice. Before proceeding with this, however, the cantilever on the opposite side should be examined for the same fault. If this is also inadequate then the framework will have to be re— made.

Fractured complete overdentures are almost invariably caused by the weakening effect of providing space within the denture for the implants and retention system. Apart from thickening the denture which is usually undesirable, the best remedy is to incorporate a thin cobalt—chromium plate in the lingual flange. To ensure the most effective strengthening effect this should be of greater overall width than the contained implant and retention parts.

FRACTURED OVERDENTURE CLIPS

Isolated fractures may be due to patient mishandling, but a repeated fracture or loosening of clips should be taken as a

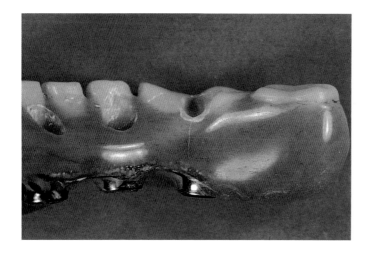

Fig 12-2 a *Lingual hair–line crack in denture base.*

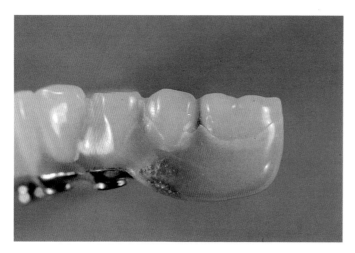

Fig 12-2 b *Visibly short cantilever supporting a larger occlusal table.*

clear signal that a problem exists elsewhere.

Horizontal denture movements in function, clip to bar misalignments, over tensioned clips, and clips fitted to curved bar parts can singly or collectively contribute to failure. Clips should only be replaced once. If the failure re–occurs a complete revision of the retention system and occlusion of the teeth should be made.

Fractured clips and curved bars

Depending on the displaceability of the underlying soft tissues, overdentures under occlusal load find their own clip to bar axis of rotation. If the bar is curved, then clips cannot form a single rotational axis. As one clip is able to correctly rotate on its part of the bar, others must deform in an attempt to comply (Figs 12-3 a and b).

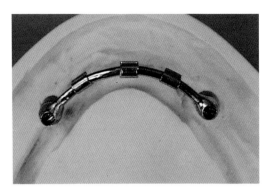

Fig 12-3 a *Curved overdenture bar with attached broken clips.*

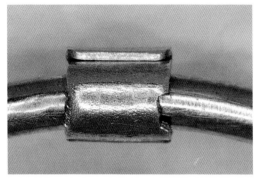

Fig 12-3 b *Clips break away from the denture by fracture of their retention tags. Compare broken clip remnant with Fig 12-4 a.*

Clips fractured under these circumstances are not dealt with adequately if they are only replaced. The only satisfactory solution is to remake the bar with a main straight part which is as near as possible at right angles to the median line and confine the clips to this part of the bar (Fig 12-3 c). Clip to bar functional misalignments are exacerbated when accompanied by horizontal movements arriving from unstable lower dentures (see Chapter 9). These movements can be very destructive. If unstable overdentures are found to have their last molar teeth set over steeply inclined residual ridge parts this may well be the seat of the problem. The dentist will check this by removing the bar from the mouth before loading the occlusal surfaces of the last molar teeth and comparing the effect of this with pressure on the first molar teeth. Offending teeth can be removed by grinding and the denture re—polished. It must be possible for the dentist to apply occlusal pressure from a finger tip or hand instrument on any artificial tooth without denture movement. When occlusal balance has not been provided, the dentures should be either correctly ground—in or remade.

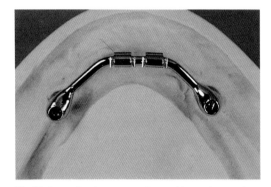

Fig 12-3 c *Replacement bar with main straight and angled subsidiary parts. Note new position of clips.*

Nobelpharma Overdenture Kit type DCA 110 (Rounded clips and wrought bar)

Some of these bars have a 2.10 mm diameter, which requires a deliberately hard polishing to achieve the design diameter of 2 mm. Great care is needed to do this successfully. The clips provided for this bar are similar to those made by the Cendres & Metaux Company and are still used by them for a 1.90 mm diameter wrought bar which they manufacture (Fig 9-9).

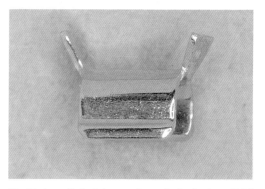

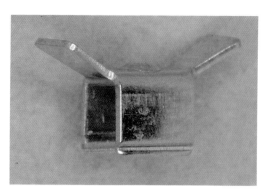

Fig 12-4 a *Nobelpharma 'rounded' clip type DCA 078.*

Fig 12-4 b *Nobelpharma 'square' clip type DCA 078.*

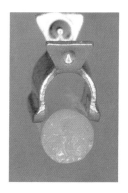
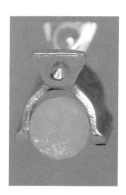

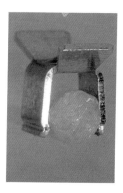

Fig 12-5 a (left) *Nobelpharma rounded clip resting on a 2.25 mm diameter plastic pattern.*

Fig 12-5 b (right) *Nobelpharma rounded clip forced onto a 2.25 mm diameter bar.*

Fig 12-5 c (below) *Nobelpharma square clip forced onto a 2.25 mm diameter bar springs upward under its own tension.*

Nobelpharma Overdenture Kit type DCA 130 (Rectangular clips and plastic pattern for a cast bar)

If retainer clips attached to this cast bar break, the diameter of the bar may be incorrectly large. This should be the first thing to be checked.

These bars and their accompanying clips fall into two types, an earlier bar supplied with rounded clips (Fig 12-4 a), and more recent ones with squarer clips (Fig 12-4 b). Both types of bar have the same Nobelpharma type number, DCA 130.

For some time these plastic patterns have been inadvertently supplied with a 2.25 mm diameter instead of the stated 2.00 mm. The supplied clip is intended for use with both the wrought bar, which has a diameter of 2.00 mm and the oversized cast bar. Neither the earlier rounded clip or later squarer clip can be fitted on the 2.25 mm diameter plastic bar unless it is distorted to place (Figs 12-5 a–c).

Clip problem 1

If a rounded clip fractures or becomes

loose, the diameter of the bar must be checked and must be 2.00 mm. If the bar diameter is correct and no denture instability problems are found, the clip may be replaced with either a rounded or rectangular clip. If the bar is measured to be 2.25 mm in diameter it must be replaced, no clip will correctly fit it.

Clip problem 2

If the rectangular clip fractures or becomes loose, its cast bar is likely to be a 2.25 mm diameter one. In this event it must be replaced with a bar of correct diameter. Only if the reader is very confident will an attempt be made to reduce the oversized bar to a perfectly round 2 mm diameter by grinding and polishing. When a correctly sized bar has been provided the failed clip is then replaced with either the rounded or rectangular type. It is not always easy to distinguish between wrought and cast bars. For this reason it is careful practice to check the diameter of all overdenture bars before replacing clips.

Clip replacement

Clips are easily replaced at the chairside, by first temporarily attaching the clip to its bar with cyanoacrylate cement before applying autopolymerising resin in a recess provided in the denture. With a laboratory repair the dentist first takes an overall impression of the bar in the mouth, having previously removed undercuts with soft wax. New clips are then attached to the bar on the model and these incorporated in the denture using autopolymerising resin.

FRACTURED OVERDENTURE BARS

Cast bars are difficult to make in longer spans. The problem is one of devising a spruing system which avoids contraction porosity. Sprues attached to the bar itself are difficult to remove without causing surface defects at the site of their connection and removal. Sprues attached only to the cylinders may not be sufficiently able to feed the central bar parts without porosity. Cast bars are liable to fracture where there are surface defects and/or porosity. Bars should be made from heat strengthened type 4 gold alloy and heavy grinding and polishing avoided.

Wrought bars almost always fail at the site of a weak soldered joint (Fig 12-6). Such joints need to be strengthened as well as re—soldered.

After the broken parts have been joined together in the mouth with Dura Lay resin, the bar is embedded in soldering investment (a). In a two joint bar both joints are re—soldered, each with U shaped wire strengthening enlargement as necessary (Figs 9-11 a–c). Regardless of the melting temperature of solder used, soldering must not take place onto gold cylinders retained by gold screws. Screws are annealed and spoiled by exposure to the heat of soldering (Chapter 14).

DISTORTED AND FRACTURED FRAMEWORKS

These are serious problems. In some instances it is difficult to discover the reason for failure, in others over—long cantilevers, thin and/or porous frameworks are obvious causes.

In every case of framework failure the

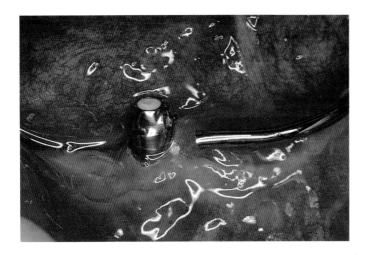

Fig 12-6 *Fractured overdenture bar to gold cylinder soldered joint. Note small area of attachment.*

internal parts of gold cylinders should be examined under magnification. The machined internal surfaces of cylinders can record much of their thermal history and possible abuse. Casting alloy overheating can produce a range of cylinder deteriorations, ranging from a partial loss of detail, through to a complete meltdown (Fig 5-7c and Fig 10-2). When gold cylinder fitting surface damage is combined with framework fracture there is no alternative but to remake everything.

Distorted frameworks

These fall into two groups: those which were originally fitted in a distorted condition and those which have permanently deformed in use. The former is often accompanied by rapid bone loss and this may be how the clinician discovered the problem. The latter is revealed by the fracture of teeth and/or denture base. Nothing can be done with frameworks which are distorted overall. Alternatively, if the framework accurately fits the implants but a cantilever has deformed, then this may be

due to an inadequate cantilever dimension for the strength of alloy used. In the event of cantilever replacement, this must be made stronger. If both cantilevers have distorted and/or other framework parts are assessed as flimsy, nothing can be done about this.

Fractured frameworks

The most common site for failure is the area where a cantilever joins a gold cylinder, since this is where the major strain occurs (Chapter 5).

If a heat strengthened type 4 gold alloy with the correct dimensions has been used the fracture will almost certainly be due to porosity, a problem which closely attends poor sprue design and alloy overheating. Poor design is also a factor, in that either the recommended sprue diameter has been used with an enlarged framework or alternatively, a framework of the correct dimensions has been cast with sprues which are too narrow (Figs 12-7a–d).

Whether to repair a broken framework

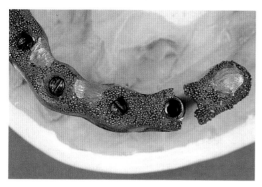

Fig 12-7 a *Fractured type 4 gold alloy cantilever of apparently robust construction. The broken cantilever is only 10 mm long.*

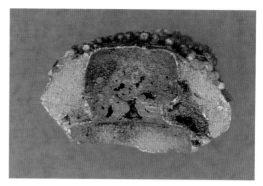

Fig 12-7 b *Porosity in cantilever fragment fracture face. The framework is over 7 mm wide at this point which is too large for the 4 mm sprue diameter apparently used.*

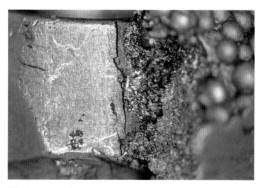

Fig 12-7 c *Cantilever gold cylinder situated in the fracture face showing its own crack.*

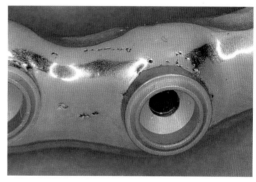

Fig 12-7 d *Contraction porosity beneath a 4 mm diameter sprue in a framework of enlarged dimensions.*

when other parts show porosity or are too thin is a difficult decision. One may be inclined to remake in these circumstances, which is a safe option.

Frameworks are frequently found to be ill fitting as well as fractured.

When the prosthesis with the fractured cantilever shown in Figs 12-8 a and b was connected to its master cast with a single screw in the patients left cantilever implant, various perpendicular discrepancy gaps were visible elsewhere. Similarly, when the fractured and almost new pros-

thesis shown in Fig 12-8 c was connected to its master cast using all the gold screws, an excellent fitting was observed. Upon removing all the screws except one in the patients right cantilever implant, the true vertical and horizontal fitting errors actually applying were then revealed (Fig 12-8 d). Also disclosed was that the archived model and its contained abutment replicas were additionally inaccurate (Fig 12-8 e). Both prostheses failed because of extensive framework porosity.

Alternatively, if the fit of a broken frame-

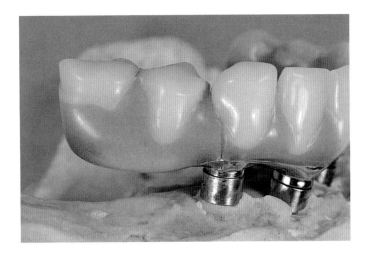

Fig 12-8 a *Fractured cantilever temporarily replaced for photography. Framework misfitting revealed by a single fixing screw placed in the patients left cantilever implant.*

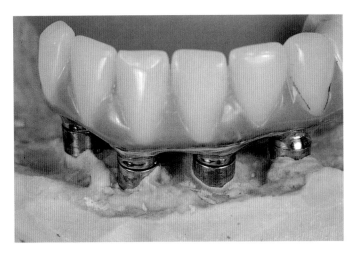

Fig 12-8 b *Easily seen perpendicular framework fitting errors.*

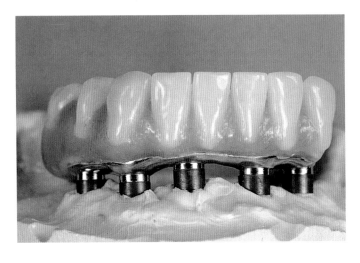

Fig 12-8 c *New prosthesis with fractured left cantilever showing an excellent fitting when all screws are in place.*

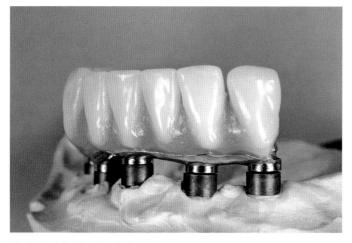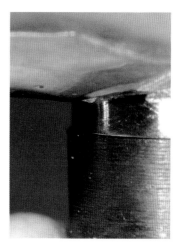

Fig 12-8 d (left) *Vertical and horizontal misfitting with a single gold screw in the patients right cantilever implant.*

Fig 12-8 e (right) *Detail of horizontal fitting error in faulty abutment replica with single gold screw tightened in place.*

work in the mouth and on an accurate archived model is satisfactory, a cantilever repair may be considered, with strengthening corrections as necessary. Unsatisfactory will be the position of the soldered joint exactly at the site of the original fracture and in the position of maximum strain (Fig 12-7 a). Gold cylinders are usually in the fracture face and contain one or more fine cracks as a result (Fig 12-7 c); an additional weakness which confirms that a soldered joint repair must not be made here.

It has been shown that functional stresses resolved in frameworks for edentulous jaws are much less in those parts removed from cantilevers (Chapter 5). With this in mind the broken framework is divided with a slanting cut to remove the cantilever gold cylinder and its immediate neighbour. The angled cut has the effect of increasing the surface area and therefore strength of the soldered joint (Fig 12-9 a). The metal forming the discarded

part of the framework can usually be used again, providing the gold cylinders are removed. This is most easily achieved by individually removing the cylinders with tweezers as the fragment is flame melted.

A new cantilever and part framework of the correct dimensions, incorporating two new gold cylinders, is made in type 4 gold alloy (Figs 12-9 b and c). After taking care not to re-introduce lateral fitting errors from inaccurate replicas (Figs 12-9 d and e), the new framework part is soldered to what remains of the original casting. By this design the soldered joint is removed to a position of low stress.

Depending on the solder used, the framework must be heat strengthened in accordance with the alloy manufacturers instructions before polishing and used again in a new prosthesis (Fig 12-9 f).

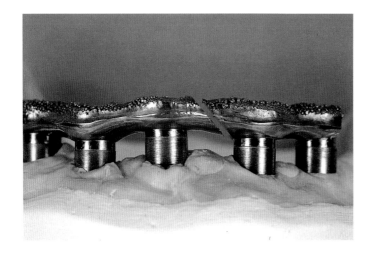

Fig 12-9 a *Framework divided with a slanting cut.*

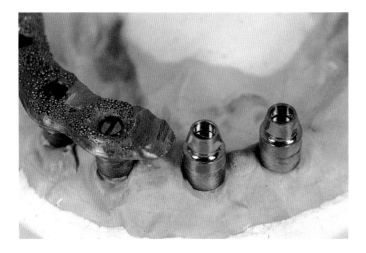

Fig 12-9 b *Two new gold cylinders will be included in the repair.*

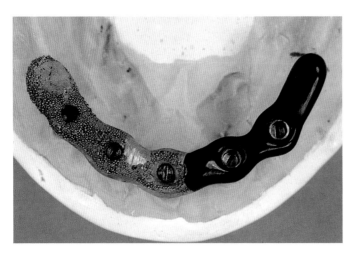

Fig 12-9 c *A Dura Lay resin repair sub-frame covered with inlay wax.*

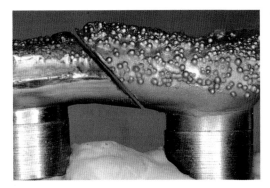 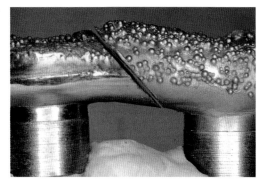

Fig 12-9 d (left) *Master cast containing faulty replicas allowing a misfitting of the new cantilever.*

Fig 12-9 e (right) *Correctly adjusted position of the cantilever on the abutment replica.*

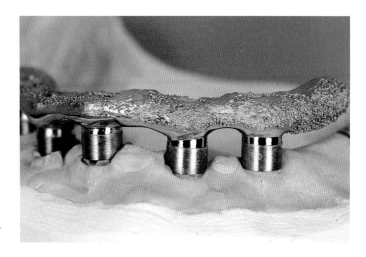

Fig 12-9 f *Completed strengthened repair.*

BROKEN GOLD SCREWS

Despite their correct pre—load tensioning, a precursor to fracture failure is often the loosening of screws in function.

The need for screw re—tightening will be regarded by the dentist as an indication that problems of occlusion, prosthesis overhang (Fig 3-8 b) and misfitting may exist. Screw fracture confirms this fact. When correctly used gold screws are strong, fatigue resistant and should not be replaced until the reasons for failure have been found and corrected. In searching for likely causal errors prostheses should be checked for fit in the mouth using the Sheffield one screw test, followed by a laboratory assessment of framework design and manufacture, and occlusion of the teeth.

In the past Nobelpharma screws with internal hexagon (part DCA 074) would occasionally fail on correct tightening or after short periods of use in the mouth

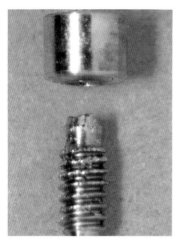

Fig 12-10 a *Gold screw fractured during correct tightening.*

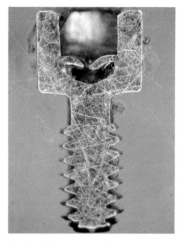

Fig 12-10 b *Sectioned screw showing weak connection of head with threaded shank.*

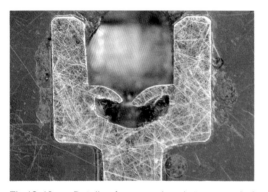

Fig 12-10 c *Detail of screw head to threaded shank construction.*

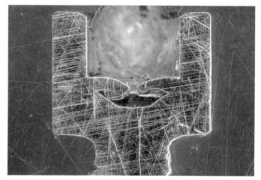

Fig 12-10 d *Gold screw of stronger construction.*

(Figs 12-10 a–c). Using finite element analysis, Sheffield University research determined that fracture in this case was due to an inadequate web of metal provided at the neck of the screw. The re—designed replacement, which has the same part number, is now satisfactorily stronger (Fig 12-10 d).

THE REPAIR OF PROSTHESES CONTAINING OBSOLETE PARTS

Older prosthetic parts from several different manufacturers have been discontinued and have been replaced by other non—interchangeable components. Obsolescent Nobelpharma parts for the Brånemark implant are still available to special order and Nobelpharma (UK) Ltd, has

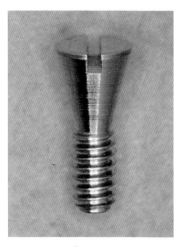

Fig 12-11 a   *Conical gold screw.*

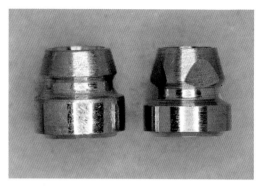

Fig 12-11 b   *Conical gold cylinder (left) and current gold cylinder (right).*

indicated that the Company intends to continue to manufacture these parts in the foreseeable future.

The use of discontinued parts needs description if prostheses are to be properly maintained and repaired.

Conical gold screws (Part DCA 014) and matching cylinders (Part DCA 013)

Conical screws were discontinued because of a loss of screw tightening energy from friction in their tapered head on tightening (Figs 12-11 a and b).[2] These parts are not interchangeable with current gold cylinders, so screw replacements must again be conical.

When framework repairs require the use of guide pins, conical guide pins DCA 027 (10 mm), DCA 053 (15 mm) and DCA 054 (20 mm) are also necessary. If frameworks containing conical cylinders have to be re—made the more efficient flat headed screws and matching gold cylinders may be substituted. These parts

accurately fit the earlier titanium abutments.

Single tooth abutment (Abutments DCA 085 to DCA 089)

For the purposes of repair and maintenance this abutment has the advantage of easy clinical retrievability, in that the crown and its abutment complete is removed from the mouth by the removal of an accessible abutment screw.

The abutment has a collar height of between 1 mm and 5 mm and consists of a titanium hexagon which becomes cylindrical as it emerges towards the incisal edge (Fig 12-12). If these crowns have to be altered because of soft tissue recession and abutment exposure, a new abutment with a shorter collar will be required. Under these circumstances the clinician may choose to replace the abutment and crown complete with the more recent CeraOne single tooth derivation.

When the abutment is satisfactory its

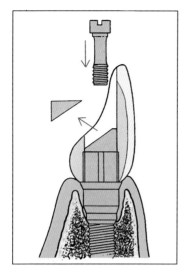

Fig 12-12 *The single tooth abutment showing its constituent parts and cemented crown. The abutment can be ground to alter its shape relative to the opposing teeth (arrowed). The crown has a single fixing/abutment screw.*

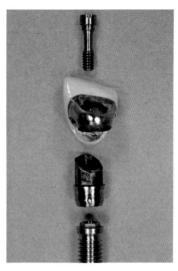

Fig 12-13 a *Parts comprising the single tooth restoration. From above, the abutment screw, metal–ceramic crown, single tooth abutment and the fixture.*

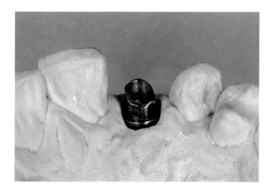

Fig 12-13 b *Abutment in place on archived cast.*

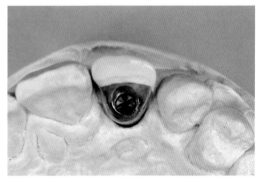

Fig 12-13 c *Completed new crown ready for cementation onto the abutment followed by connection to the fixture by means of the abutment screw.*

crown can be altered or re—made as required. With metal—ceramic crowns a new coping is then cast and porcelain added as necessary. Light—cured composite materials may be conveniently formed directly onto the abutment cylinder (Figs 12-13 a–c).

REFERENCES

1. Strid K-G. Chapter 11, Radiographic Results. Tissue-Integrated Prostheses, Osseointegration in Clinical Dentistry 1987 [Brånemark P-I, Zarb G A, Albrektsson T]. Quintessence Publishing Co, Inc, Chicago, USA.

2. Jorneus L. Screws and cylinders in the Nobelpharma implant system. *Nobelpharma News* 1987; 1: 7.

CHAPTER 12: MATERIALS AND EQUIPMENT

Manufacturer	UK Distributor
(a) Deguvest L soldering investment	
Degussa AG	Degussa Limited
Postfach 110533	Winterton House
D-6000 Frankfurt 11	Winterton Way
Germany	Macclesfield
	SK11 0LP

Chapter Thirteen
Treatment Consequences

For those of us who have our own natural teeth we cannot really know what it is to have lost teeth and be suffering for it. Patients in this situation cannot easily express the feelings they have, especially to members of the dental team. With this difficulty in mind the Sheffield Dental School has always arranged for those seeking treatment to meet and talk with people who have already received implants. The interaction can be quite amazing.

Restoring secure and efficient teeth is only part of a solution. Implants can provide much more than this. Those who have to wear conventional dentures (or indeed spectacles or hearing aids) can never fully accept them as part of themselves; or as part of the persona. By contrast, patients with fixed implant supported prostheses appear to accept that they have been provided with something which is part of themselves. Many will use such phrases as "I only remember that I have implants when I come to see you!". When this is so, the prospect of prostheses removal for any reason even temporarily, is regarded with total dismay.

Reports have also shown that the psychological consequences of providing patients with implants can be quite dramatic. However, written reports and patients' personal comments are but poor vehicles to convey what is really happening. Some measure of what has taken place can perhaps be detected in the accompanying illustrations.

In addition to severe problems of denture function the patient shown in Fig 13-1 was unhappy with her appearance.

Using the same make and mould of teeth as originally supplied, new complete upper and implant supported overdenture lower dentures were provided (Fig 13-2). These were tried—in and the patients opinion sought (Fig 13-3). One month after the dentures were placed the patient returned for assessment (Fig 13-4).

The appearance of the teeth is self evident and is not difficult to achieve. In comparing the patients previous and final appearance, ignore the teeth. Look instead at the hair, the way that the muscles of the cheeks and lips fall in place, and especially look at the eyes.

The dental implant team at the University of Sheffield Dental School, like others throughout the world, do not really know what it is that osseointegrated dental technology gives these patients, but whatever it is, it's wonderful.

Ars Longa Vita Brevis

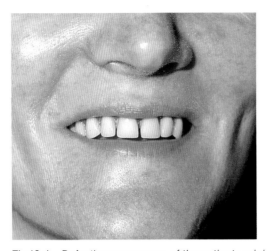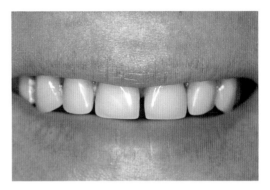

Fig 13-1   *Defective appearance of the patients original complete dentures.*

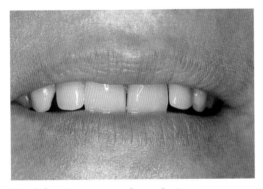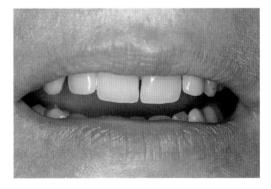

Fig 13-2   *Appearance of new dentures.*

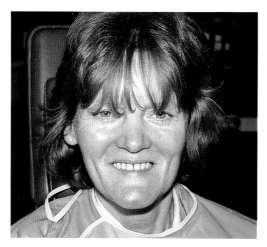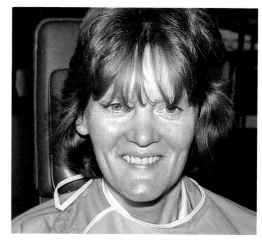

Fig 13-3 *Try—in of dentures. (Left) the old ones, (right) the new implant supported ones.*

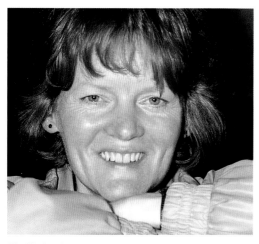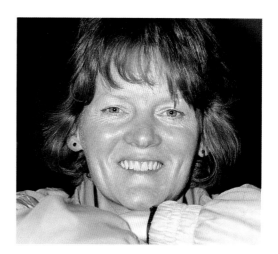

Fig 13-4 *Patients appearance one month later.*

Chapter Fourteen
Technical Data

The author has found that a file of accurate technical data on components and materials is an invaluable aid to laboratory work.

The data file presented in this chapter has been compiled by the author for his own use and thus reflects very much the components and material which are regularly used in his own laboratory.

Other laboratories will wish to compile their own data file to meet their own needs and the author would strongly recommend that they do this.

This data file has been compiled from information provided by manufacturers who are usually only too willing to supply necessary information.

Abutment Replicas
Nobelpharma

Replica for the standard abutment (Brass)	DCB 015
Replica for the EsthetiCone and Angulated abutment (Brass)	DCB 105
Replica for the CeraOne abutment (Plastic)	DCA 129

Casting Alloys
Stabilor G

Type	4, Extra Hard

Composition (%)

Gold	58.00
Silver	23.3.
Base metals	13.0
Melting range (°C)	860–940

Vickers hardness

a) annealed	170
b) hardened	275
c) slow cooled after casting	275

Ultimate tensile strength (N/mm^2)

a) annealed	510
b) slow cooled after casting	890

0.2 % Yield strength (N/mm^2)

a) annealed	400
b) slow cooled after casting	830

Elongation (%)

a) annealed	33
b) slow cooled after casting	6
Density (g/cm^3)	14.4

Matticraft E

Type	Metal–ceramic

Composition (%)

Gold	17.6
Silver	1.1
Platinum	9.6
Palladium	8.6

Melting Range (°C)	1180–1240
Casting Temperature (°C)	1290–1390
Mould Temperature (°C)	850

Mechanical properties

Vickers Hardness	175
Elongation (%)	6
Tensile Strength (N/mm^2)	635

Herabond E

Type	Metal–ceramic

Composition (%)

Gold	45.00
Palladium	32.00
Silver	18.00

Melting Range (°C)	1220–1280
Casting Temperature (°C)	1430
Mould Temperature (°C)	850
Recommended crucible	graphite
Annealing (°C)	5 minutes at 950
Hardening (°C)	15 minutes at 650

Mechanical properties

Hardness (DIN 13906)	(Annealed)	205
	(Hardened)	240
Elongation (%)	(Annealed)	13
	(Hardened)	9
Density (g/cm^2)		14.0

Gold Cylinders

Standard cylinders and Conical gold cylinders for the Angulated Abutment

Nobelpharma Parts DCA 072, DCA 073, DCA 103

Composition (%)

Gold	10.0
Platinum	39.5
Palladium	26.0
Silver	24.5
Density (g/mm^3)	14.6
Melting range (°C)	1280–1350

Mechanical properties	*Annealed*
Vickers hardness	220
Yield strength (N/mm^2)	745
Ultimate tensile strength (N/mm^2)	1000
Elongation (%)	5

Dimensions

a) Standard gold cylinders

Height (mm) (DCA 073)	3.0
Height (mm) (DCA 072)	4.0

b) Tapered gold cylinder (DCA 103)

Height (mm)	5.7
Height overall when attached to 4.0×1.5 mm Angulated abutment (mm)	8.5
Height overall when attached to 5.5×3.0 mm Angulated abutment (mm)	10.0

It is not possible to harden these cylinders (Nobelpharma AB, personal communication, 1991).

Gold Cylinders, EsthetiCone

Nobelpharma Part DCA 141

Composition (%)

Gold	10.5
Platinum	39.5
Palladium	36.0
Silver	14.4
Density (g/mm^3)	14.7
Melting range (°C)	1460–1500

Mechanical properties	*Annealed*	*Hardened*
Vickers hardness	234	286
Yield strength (N/mm^2)	650	750
Ultimate tensile strength (N/mm^2)	700	790
Elongation (%)	6	4
Hardening (°C)	30 mins at 700	

Dimension

Height (mm)	5.7

Gold Cylinder for CeraOne Abutment

Nobelpharma Part DCA 160

Dimensions (mm)

Height	5.10
Width of cylinder	4.40
Overall width	4.80

Gold Screws

Nobelpharma Parts DCA 074, DCA 075

Composition (%)

Gold	61.40
Platinum	12.70
Silver	16.40
Copper	9.10
Palladium	0.20

Iridium	0.10
Zinc	0.10

Mechanical properties

Hardened

Ultimate tensile strength (N/mm^2)	880
Yield stress (N/mm^2)	830
Elongation (%)	14
Hardness (Hv)	230

Annealed

Ultimate tensile strength (N/mm^2)	685
Yield stress (N/mm^2)	490
Elongation (%)	30
Hardness (Hv)	151

Gold Solders

for Dolder Bar joints and Articulated Retention Grip Bars

Melting point (°C)	
S.G2	825
S.G3	740

Herador
For pre–ceramic soldering of Herabond E

Herador Lot 0. Melting point (°C)	1100
Herador Lot 1. Melting point (°C)	1060

For post–ceramic soldering of Herabond E

Herador Lot 2. Melting point (°C)	800

Head Screws

Type	Thread diam (mm)	Thread length (mm)	Screw head height/diam (mm)	Total length screw/sleeve (mm)	Sleeve diam (mm)
143.08.2	0.80	1.40	3.80/1.30	6.00	1.40
143.08.5	0.80	2.40	3.80/1.30	7.00	1.40
143.10.2	1.00	1.70	3.80/1.50	6.40	1.60
143.10.5	1.00	3.40	3.80/1.50	8.10	1.60
143.12.2	1.20	1.90	3.80/1.70	6.60	1.80
143.12.5	1.20	3.90	3.80/1.70	8.60	1.80
143.14.2	1.40	2.40	4.20/2.10	7.60	2.00
143.14.5	1.40	4.40	4.20/2.10	9.60	2.00
143.16.2	1.60	2.60	4.40/2.50	8.00	2.20
143.16.5	1.60	4.90	4.40/2.50	10.30	2.20

Healing Caps
Nobelpharma

Healing cap plastic 4.5 mm
diameter   DCA 045

Obsolete Components
Nobelpharma

a. Tapered gold screw and cylinder

a) Conical (tapered) gold
   screws   DCA 014
b) Conical gold cylinder
   (4 mm)   DCA 013

b. Single tooth abutments
Fixture replica   DCA 084

Abutments

a) 1 mm   DCA 085
b) 2 mm   DCA 086
c) 3 mm   DCA 087
d) 4 mm   DCA 088
e) 5 mm   DCA 089

Overdenture Retainer Type I
**Nobelpharma Overdenture Kit
with wrought gold bar**   DCA 110

Comprising

One gold bar, 30 mm long,
2 mm diameter   DCA 077
Two gold cylinders (4 mm)   DCA 072
Two gold screws   DCA 075
Two clip attachments and
spacers   DCA 078

Dimensions (mm)

Spacer thickness   0.75
Overall height of bar,
spacer and clip attachments   4.10
Width of clip and bar   2.60

**Nobelpharma Overdenture Kit
with plastic pattern bar**   DCA 130

Comprising

One plastic bar, 30 mm long,
2 mm diameter   DCA 079
Two gold cylinders (4 mm)   DCA 072

Two gold screws   DCA 075
Two clip attachments and
spacers   DCA 078

Dimensions
As wrought bar.

Dolder Bar Joint
Dimensions (mm)

Maximum bar length available	200
Maximum sleeve length	50
Lengths available	
(Bar and sleeve complete)	20, 30, 50

Dolder bar joints are available in two cross-sectional sizes, Numbers 53.01.2 and 53.01.5

Dolder 53.01.2

Dimensions (mm)

Height bar, sleeve and spacer	3.50
Bar width	1.60
Sleeve width	2.10
Sleeve retention width	3.50
Maximum vertical movement	
before loss of function	0.75
Sleeve activating tool, part	51.01.25
Sleeve deactivator tool, part	51.01.255

Dolder 53.01.5

Height bar, sleeve and spacer	4.55
Bar width	2.20
Sleeve width	2.80
Sleeve retention width	4.50
Maximum vertical movement	
before loss of function	1.05
Sleeve activating tool, part	51.01.25
Sleeve deactivator tool, part	51.01.555

Articulated Retention Grip Bars
CM Bar 55.01.2

Dimensions (mm)

Bar lengths available	50, 100, 200
Diameter of	1.90
Overall height of bar, rider	
and spacer	2.75
Length of rider	3.50
Maximum vertical movement	
before loss of function	0.50
Bar lengths available	50, 100, 200
Rider activating tool, part	51.01.25

After soldering, the bar is strengthened by furnace heating at 400 °C for 15 min.

Overdenture Retainer Type II
Nobelpharma Ball Attachment DCA 114
Comprising

Two plastic caps each with	
resilient O-ring	DCA 113
Two spacers	DCA 112
Two ball attachment replicas	DCA 111

Dimensions (mm)

Width of cap	7.20
Height of cap	5.50
Spacer height	0.60

Protection Caps
Nobelpharma

For standard gold cylinders	DCB 092
For conical gold cylinders	DCA 143

Retention Cylinders, Temporary

Implant Innovations   Type TRC 30

For Brånemark and IMZ implant systems.

Screwdrivers

Nobelpharma

For gold screws with slot

37 mm	DIB 047
75 mm	DIB 046

For gold screws with hexagon

37 mm	DIB 172
75 mm	DIB 171

Temporary Components

Nobelpharma

Temporary cylinder for standard abutments	DCA 159
Temporary cylinder for EsthetiCone and Angulated abutments	DCA 157

Dimensions (mm)

Height	12.00
Height after reduction for Tube connection	6.20

Height of resulting cone	5.00
Width at skirt	5.30
Height of skirt	1.50
Temporary Tube	DCA 158

Dimensions (mm)

Height	10.60
Height of internal cone	5.00
Width	10.60

Temporary Cap for CeraOne abutment	DCA 161

Dimensions (mm)

Overall height (including retention elements)	15.80
Width	4.80

Vacuum Forming Material

Biocryl

Article number	3150/1
Thickness (mm)	1.5
Diameter (mm)	125
Heating time (sec)	45
Colour	clear

Index

A

Abutment replica
Angulated   98, 99
Ball attachment   166
CeraOne plastic   188, 191, 192
Damaged   108, 123, 203
For resin processing   108, 145
Inaccurate 80–82, 85–87, 90, 203, 213, 215

Abutment titanium   20, 21
Cleaning access   31, 111, 171, 203, 204
Protection of   103, 104

Angulated abutments   37, 44, 166, 169
Contra indications   98, 190

Archiving   108, 133, 151, 167, 203, 211, 213

B

Bone
As a bed for implants   61, 62–66
Assessment for cantilever length   111
Damaging stresses in   61, 75–91, 200
Healing time   39, 62
Loads resolved in   63–66
Loss   78, 85, 203, 210
Quality of   39, 62
Remodelling   47, 48
Safe loading of   48, 61, 62
Shape of as overdenture foundations   153–157

C

Cantilevers
Anteriorly projecting   179–182
Clearance from soft tissues   111, 203, 204
Dimensions of   61, 111, 113, 171
Distorted   209, 210
Fatigue endurance and strength of   72–74
Fracture and repair   210–215
Loads transmitted by   63–66, 76

Cap
Healing   103, 104, 154
Polishing protection   53, 54, 124, 147
Temporary   58, 59

Casting
Mould cooling interval   121
Temperature accuracy   67–70

Casting alloys
Amount necessary   120
Choice of   70, 171, 172
Cooling contraction   71, 72
Heat treatment strengthening   72, 121, 123
Overheating   67, 68–71
Porosity   164, 209–211
Superheating   67, 70, 72

Casting investments
Choice of   67, 71, 72, 78, 118, 176
Deterioration of   78, 118
Expansion   71, 72, 78–80
Heating   78, 118–120
Setting time   118, 119

Casting mould
Cooling distortion 121
Mould position when casting 117, 121

Complications
Abutment screw fracture 83–85
CeraOne crowns 189–192
Metal–ceramic CeraOne crowns 190–192
Gold cylinder melting 70, 71, 171
Gold screw fracture 83, 85, 86, 88, 215, 216
Horizontal framework misfitting 78–80
Implant fracture 83–85, 203
Inaccurate abutment replicas 90, 91, 211, 213
Lateral bone loading 82–88, 199, 200
Overdentures 153, 159, 164, 166, 205–210
Perpendicular framework misfitting 75–77, 80
Screw access hole position 95, 96

D

Dentures opposing implant supported prostheses
Canine replacement 135–138
Reduced occlusal table 134–138
Stability of 134–138, 153–157

F

Fitting prostheses
Compound 178, 179
EsthetiCone prostheses 199, 200
Fixed prostheses 149, 150

Fixed maxillary prostheses
Angulated abutments for 169
Anterior cantilevers 179–181
Cantilever length 171
Metal–ceramic prostheses 171, 197–200

Prostheses with resin teeth 169, 170, 193–195

Framework
Anterior cantilevers 179–182
Causes of horizontal fitting errors 78–80
Causes of perpendicular errors 79–80, 120
Design considerations 61–66
Dimensions 111, 113
Fitting accuracy 61, 75, 76, 78–80, 123, 124, 127, 129
Function and requirements for 22, 61, 62
Metal–ceramic 171, 172, 197
Misfitting stressing of implants and bone 75–78, 83–86
Records of 126, 127
Weight of 120, 121

G

Gold cylinders 20, 21
Cast metal on fitting surface 80, 123, 124
For CeraOne abutment 191, 192
For EsthetiCone abutment 172, 195
Polishing caps for 124, 147
Thermal damage 67, 70, 71, 171, 172

Gold screw access hole difficulties 95, 96, 169

Gold screws
Fracture 65, 66, 83–86, 88
Function 61
Loosening 65, 66, 85, 215, 216
Settling 66
Stressing 64–67, 74, 83, 85, 200
Tightening 66–67, 85

Guide pins
In impressions 104–108
Removal from prostheses 146, 147
Shortening 141, 143

H

Heat treatment strengthening
Overdenture bars 162, 163
Problems of 77, 90
Type 4 gold alloy frameworks 72, 123

I

Implants
As load bearing foundations 20, 22, 24, 61–63
Stresses from prostheses 75–77, 80–87, 199, 200
Healing time 39
Number needed 36
Patients do not want implants 24
Positions of 37, 43, 44, 61, 95–97, 169, 186
Survival rates 23
Technical significance of fixture loss 44

Implant dental technology
As part of a team 25, 90
Objectives 24, 25

Investment
Choice of 67, 71, 72, 78, 176
Deterioration of 78, 118
Effect of expansion on moulds 80
Setting time 118

M

Misfitting prostheses
Corrective soldering 77, 78, 85, 86
Fitting criteria 61, 75, 76, 85, 86
Implant screw failure 83–85, 86, 88
Sprue induced misfitting 120
Perpendicular errors 75–79

O

Overdentures
Clip fracture 153, 154, 159, 164, 205–207, 208
Functional stability of 153–158, 207
Overdenture fracture 205
Setting–up for 156–158

P

Partial prostheses
Accurate fixture placement 186, 196–198
Advantages 185
CeraOne crowns 186–190
EsthetiCone abutments, space for 196, 197
Prostheses with resin teeth 193–195

Provisional prostheses
Advantages of 38, 47, 48
Temporary frameworks 57, 58

R

Resin teeth 156, 169, 170
Advantages of 133, 193–195
Screw access holes in 134, 140–143, 148

S

Screw access holes, unsightly 95, 96

Setting–up
Canine/premolar substitution 135–138
Overdenture stability 153–158
Reduced occlusal table 135, 138

Sheffield fitting test 61, 85, 123, 174
Sheffield wax strip test 127, 129
Overdenture bars 164

T

Treatment objectives 61

Treatment planning 31